Practical Pharmaceutical Chemistry (II) and VIVA VOCE

Second Edition

for Diploma in Pharmacy and
B Pharmacy Students

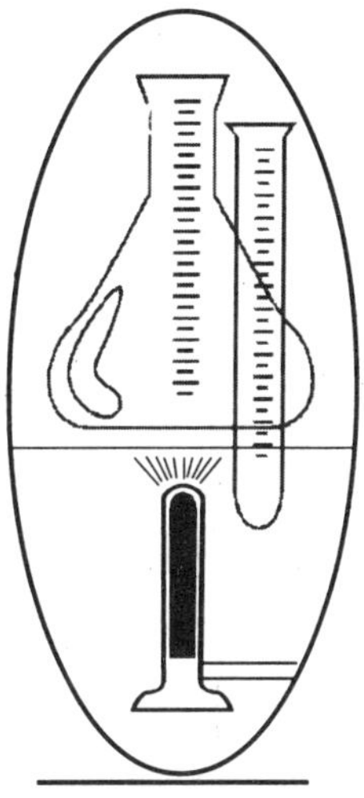

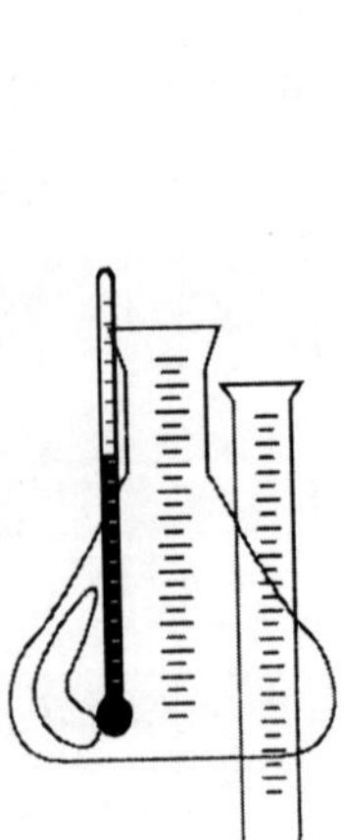

Practical Pharmaceutical Chemistry (II) and VIVA VOCE

Second Edition

for Diploma in Pharmacy and B Pharmacy Students

NIRMAL SHARMA MPharm, PhD, FICN, AIC

Young Investigator's Award Winner 1993 and Member of International Board of Research Studies selected by the American Biographical Institute

Assistant Professor
Department of Pharmacognosy and Phytochemistry
Delhi Institute of Pharmaceutical Sciences and Research
Pushp Vihar, Sector -3, New Delhi - 110017

YOGESHWAR SHARMA PhD
Associate Professor, Department of Applied Chemistry
Debub University, Awassa, Ethiopia

G.C. SHARMA PhD
Lecturer (Selection Grade), Department of Chemistry
Narmada College of Science and Commerce
Zadeshwar, Bharuch

CBSPD

CBS Publishers & Distributors Pvt Ltd

New Delhi • Bengaluru • Chennai • Kochi • Kolkata • Lucknow • Mumbai
Hyderabad • Jharkhand • Nagpur • Patna • Pune • Uttarakhand

Disclaimer

Science and technology are constantly changing fields. New research and experience broaden the scope of information and knowledge. The authors have tried their best in giving information available to them while preparing the material for this book. Although, all efforts have been made to ensure optimum accuracy of the material, yet it is quite possible some errors might have been left uncorrected. The publisher, the printer and the authors will not be held responsible for any inadvertent errors or inaccuracies.

Practical Pharmaceutical Chemistry (II) and Viva Voce

ISBN: 978-81-239-1259-2

First Edition : 1998

Second Edition : 2005

Reprint: 2007, 2008, 2010, 2019, 2023

Published by Satish Kumar Jain and produced by Varun Jain for

CBS Publishers & Distributors Pvt Ltd

4819/XI Prahlad Street, 24 Ansari Road, Daryaganj, New Delhi 110 002, India

Ph: 011-23289259, 23266861, 23266867 Website: www.cbspd.com

Fax: 011-23243014 e-mail: delhi@cbspd.com

Corporate Office: 204 FIE, Industrial Area, Patparganj, Delhi 110 092, India

Ph: 011-4934 4934 Fax: 011-4934 4935 e-mail: publishing@cbspd.com; publicity@cbspd.com

Branches

- **Bengaluru:** Seema House 2975, 17th Cross, KR Road, Banasankari 2nd Stage, Bengaluru 560 070, Karnataka, India
  Ph: +91-80-26771678/79 Fax: +91-80-26771680 e-mail: bangalore@cbspd.com
- **Chennai:** 7, Subbaraya Street, Shenoy Nagar, Chennai 600 030, Tamil Nadu, India
  Ph: +91-44-26680620, 26681266 Fax: +91-44-42032115 e-mail: chennai@cbspd.com
- **Kochi:** 42/1325, 1326, Power House Road, Opp KSEB, Power House, Ernakulam, Kochi 682 018, India
  Ph: +91-484-4059061–65 Fax: +91-484-4059065 e-mail: kochi@cbspd.com
- **Kolkata:** 147, Hind Ceramics Compound, 1st Floor, Nilgunj Road, Belghoria, Kolkata 700 056, West Bengal, India
  Ph: +91-33-25633055–56 e-mail: kolkata@cbspd.com
- **Lucknow:** Basement, Khushnuma Complex, 7-Meerabai Marg (behind Jawahar Bhawan), Lucknow 226 001, India
  Ph: +91-522-4000032 e-mail: tiwari.lucknow@cbspd.com
- **Mumbai:** PWD Shed. Gala no. 25/26, Ramchandra Bhatt Marg, Next to JJ Hospital Gate no. 2, Opp. Union Bank of India, Noorbaug Mumbai 400 009, Maharashtra, India
  Ph: +91-22-66661880/89 e-mail: mumbai@cbspd.com

Representatives

- **Hyderabad** 0-9885175004 • **Jharkhand** 0-9811541605 • **Nagpur** 0-9421945513
- **Patna** 0-9334159340 • **Pune** 0-9923910676 • **Uttarakhand** 0-9716462459

Printed at SRK Graphics, Delhi, India

dedicated

to

Our Master Ji

Maharaj Charan Singh Ji

and

Maharaj Gurinder Singh Ji

Foreword

Organic chemistry is an essential ingredient in the education of scientists in a large range of fields, particularly in life sciences.

A career in pharmacy, an applied life science, is also becoming more and more dependent on organic chemistry. The practice of medicine now-a-days increasingly requires knowledge of the behaviour of molecules.

The present edition of the book *Practical Pharmaceutical Chemistry (II) and Viva Voce* has been thoroughly revised according to the new syllabus of the undergraduate pharmacy and B.Sc students of the Indian universities.

The entire subject matter has been divided into seven chapters. The first four chapters deal with various laboratory methods like tests for the functional groups, determination of melting and boiling points, preparation of derivatives, etc. which are used in the identification of the organic compounds. Chapter 5 has been thoroughly revised and now includes tests for identification and purity of drugs like chloramphenicol and ascorbic acid. Organic preparations have been dealt in Chapter 6. Another salient feature of the book is the presentation of 'questions and answers' for viva voce examination which are given in the last chapter.

The authors have been successful in their overall objective of producing a LABORATORY MANUAL which is not only up-to-date in content and approach, but which also provides sufficient details both in theory and experimental work. This knowledge will make the students confident while actually performing various experiments.

I strongly feel that the pharmacy and BSc students will find this practical manual useful.

Dr. S.C. Hari MSc, Ph.D
Reader in Chemistry, Motilal Nehru College
(Delhi University), New Delhi - 21

Preface to Second Edition

This edition of the ***Practical Pharmaceutical Chemistry (II) and Viva Voce*** has been thoroughly revised and modified according to the syllabus of undergraduate pharmacy students (according to the PCI regulations) as well as for the BSc students.

The manual provides a systematic course material on practical aspects. It has been designed to equip the students adequately to meet the unpredictable and exciting challenges of the subject.

The subject matter of the book has been organised in the form of seven chapters.

🕮 Chapters 1 and 2 explain the identification of organic compounds and their functional group analysis.

🕮 The experimental techniques for the determination of melting and boiling points of the compounds have been explained in Chapter 3.

🕮 Chapter 4 describes the preparation of derivatives with melting points.

🕮 Chapter 5 has been modified through various identification tests of the undergraduate syllabus. The additional identification tests and tests for purities for ascorbic acid, benzoic acid, chloramphenicol, caffeine and analgin according to UG syllabus have been added according to the method given in *Indian Pharmacopoeia* (1996, Volume I).

🕮 Chapter 6 on "Organic Preparations" has been updated with a number of additional experiments in the various categories of chemical reactions like :

- Oxidation–reduction reactions, specific reactions like Cemmenson–reduction, preparations of anthraquinones, etc. have been included.
- Oxime-derivative preparations have been added.

➤ Other kinds of reactions, for example esterification hydrolysis, have also been added.

➤ Besides, according to the undergraduate syllabus of B Pharmacy, specific details of electrophilic and nucleophilic substitution reactions, and various kinds of rearrangement reactions have been explained from conceptual point of view with examples.

🕮 Chapter 7 on *Viva Voce* has also been updated with additional questions on various kinds of chemical reactions.

We wish to acknowledge our greatest thanks to all those who have been associated with us for a long time for their moral encouragement. Dr. B. Subramaniam, Prof. A.K. Sharma, Dr. S.C. Hari, Dr. H.K. Saxena, Dr. N.K. Agnihotri, Dr A.M. Khan, Dr. (Mrs) Vidya Pradhan, Mrs Sharda Sushil, Dr. (Mrs) Ratan Dubey, Mrs. Ratna Chaudhary, and Mr. K.K. Thakur are thankfully acknowledged for their constant encouragement.

We are thankful to Mr. Satish K. Jain and Mr. Vinod K. Jain, CBS Publishers and Distributors, for their tireless and dynamic efforts for the publication.

Further, we are also thankful to Mr. Y.N. Arjuna, Publishing Director, CBS, for his keen interest, dedication and hard work involved in this publication.

Finally, we sincerly thank all our family members, specially Mrs. Savitri Devi Shastri, mother of Dr. Nirmal Sharma.

The first two authors, namely, Dr. Nirmal Sharma and Dr. Yogeshwar Sharma, are thankful to their loving children Richa and Lakshay, for their patience, who were neglected during the preparation of this book.

Comments and criticism from readers will be highly appreciated for improvement of their book and incorporated in the subsequent reprints and editions.

Nirmal Sharma
Yogeshwar Sharma
G.C. Sharma

Preface to First Edition

This laboratory manual of Pharmaceutical Chemistry-II has been written to meet the needs of Diploma in Pharmacy IInd year students, whose performance in Pharmaceutical Chemistry-II has been otherwise generally far from satisfactory. This poor performance is partly because of the non-availability of laboratory manual in Chemistry for diploma in pharmacy students.

This book provides a systematic course of Practical Organic Chemistry, as per education regulations-91, prescribed by Pharmacy Council of India. It is designed to equip the students adequately to meet the unpredictable and exciting challenges of the subject.

The subject matter of the book has been organized into seven Chapters. The first two chapters explain the identification of organic compounds and their tests for the functional groups. The third chapter describes the experimental techniques for determining the melting and boiling point. The fourth chapter describes the preparation of derivatives with melting points. Various identification tests for different categories of drugs have been explained in chapter five. Chapter six describes a number of preparation of compounds of synthetic, medicinal, industrial and technical importance. Simple preparations based on important name reactions, preparations involving two steps have also been included. The possible viva-voce questions with their answers from all the above mentioned chapters have been included in chapter seven.

We wish to acknowledge our greatest indebtedness to our teachers and colleagues namely Prof. J.S. Qadry, Dr. A.K. Sharma, Mrs. Kanchan Kohli, Dr. B. Subramaniam, Dr. M.R. Yadav, Dr. S.C. Hari, Dr. H.K. Saxena, Dr. S.C. Sarkar, Dr. B.S. Arora, Dr. A.M. Khan, Dr. N.K. Agnihotri, who had always been inspiring us to do something for the benefit of the profession.

We are also highly thankful to Mr. Satish Kumar Jain and Mr. Vinod Kumar Jain, CBS Publishers and Distributors for their tireless and dynamic efforts for this publication. Further we are also highly thankful to Mr. Brij Mohan Singh, Mr. Jitendra and Mr. Sen for their constant efforts for the completion of this publication.

Finally our special thanks goes to our all family members. The first two authors namely Nirmal, Yogeshwar are thankful to their loving daughter 'Richa' for her patience, whom they had neglected during their studies.

Comments and criticism from readers will be highly appreciated for improvement of this book and incorporated in subsequent editions.

New Delhi

Nirmal Sharma
Yogeshwar Sharma
G.C. Sharma

Contents

CHAPTER

1

Qualitative Organic Analysis

Qualitative organic analysis involves a series of steps that help to establish the identity of the unknown organic compound. The identification involves the following steps.

A. Preliminary Examination

Test	Observation	Inference
1. State		
	(a) Solid	Higher homologues of aromatic hydrocarbons, phenols, acids and bases may be present.
	(b) Liquid	Lower hydrocarbons, acids, amines, ketones esters, alcohols, aldehydes, etc. may be present.
2. Colour		
	(a) Colourless	Aldehydes, ketones alcohols, carbohydrates.
	(b) Yellow	Nitro compounds may be present.
	(c) Pink-brown	Aromatic amines, phenols naphthols may be present.

Test	Observation	Inference

Some examples of coloured compounds are given below:

Compound	Colour
Picric acid	Yellow
o-Nitrophenol	Yellow
m-Nitro aniline	Golden yellow
p-Nitro aniline	Pale yellow
p-Benzoquinone	Yellow
Resorcinol	Light pink
α-Naphthol	Violet
β-Naphthol	Chocolate
p-Cresol	Dark pink

3. Odour

Observation	Inference
(a) Bitter almond like	Benzaldehyde, nitrobenzene
(b) Fruity smell	Esters
(c) Spirit smell	Alcohols
(d) Fishy smell	Amines

4. Ignition Test

Test	Observation	Inference
Organic compound on a metallic spatula and ignite it over free flame	(a) Smoky flame	May be an Aromatic compound
	(b) Non-smoky flame and yellowish	May be an Aliphatic compound
	(c) Chars and leaves a black residue	May be Carbohydrates, Sugars

5. Solubility Behaviour

(i) Organic Compound + Distilled Water

Observation	Inference
(a) Completely soluble and turns blue litmus red.	Water soluble acids
(b) Completely soluble and turns red litmus blue.	Water soluble bases (lower amines)
(c) Completely soluble and neutral to lit-mus.	Neutral compounds

Test	Observation	Inference
(ii) Organic compound + 5% NaOH	Completely soluble and reappears by conc. HCl	Acids and Phenol are present

Test	Observation	Inference
(iii) Organic compound + 5% $NaHCO_3$	Organic compound dissolves with effervescence of CO_2 gas	Acid is present
(iv) Organic compound + 50% HCl	Organic compound dissolves and reappears by conc. NaOH	Base is present
6. Unsaturation Tests		
(a) Dissolve 50 mg (or 3 drops) of organic compound in 1 ml CCl_4 or acetic acid + 2% Br_2 solution dropwise.	Decolourization	+ve test for unsaturation
(b) Beyer's Test : Dissolve 50 mg (or 3 drops) of O.C. in acetone or water + 2% alkaline $KMnO_4$ soln. dropwise (1 ml of 2% $KMnO_4$ + 5 ml of 2% Na_2CO_3 soln.)	Decolourization or appearance of a soluble brown MnO_2	+ve test for unsaturation

Detection of Elements (Nitrogen, Sulphur and Halogens)

This test was introduced by J.L. Lassaigne in 1843. In this test organic compound is fused with sodium metal. The following reactions take place during fusion and convert them (N, S, X = Cl, Br, I) into water soluble salts as shown below :

$$Na + C + N \longrightarrow \underset{\text{(Sodium cyanide)}}{NaCN} \longrightarrow Na^+ + CN^-$$

$$2Na + S \longrightarrow \underset{\text{(Sodium sulphide)}}{Na_2S} \longrightarrow 2Na^+ + S^{2-}$$

$$Na + X \longrightarrow \underset{\text{(Sodium halide)}}{NaX} \longrightarrow Na^+ + X^-$$

(X = Cl, Br, I)

When nitrogen and sulphur are both present then sodium thiocyanate (sodium sulfocyanide) is formed:

$$Na + C + N + S \longrightarrow \underset{\text{(Sodium sulfocyanide)}}{NaCNS} \longrightarrow Na^+ \; CNS^-$$

Procedure

Place a small piece of freshly cut sodium metal in a dry ignition tube. The ignition tube is heated gently. Sodium melts and turns black. Remove the ignition tube from the flame and very small amount of organic compound (about 50 mg solid or 3-4 drops of liquid)* is added to it, when Immediate reaction with sodium is observed. The ignition tube is heated over a low flame for a few seconds and then it is heated strongly until the tube becomes red hot. The red hot tube is broken by immersion in 15-20 ml cold distilled water in a porcelain dish (China dish). Crush the ignition tube completely and repeat the same procedure 3-4 times. Boil the solution for 5 minutes and remove the glass splinters by filtration. The filtrate is usually called as the "Sodium fusion extract" or "Lassaigne's extract".

Test	*Observation*	*Inference*
1. Test for Nitrogen (N)		
1 ml of sodium fusion extract +1 ml of freshly	Green or prussian	'N' is present

* Instead of adding liquid alone, the paste of liquid in anhydrous sodium carbonate powder and zinc dust can be introduced in the ignition tube.

Test	*Observation*	*Inference*
prepared $FeSO_4$ solution + NaOH soln. Green ppt. are obtained, boil for 30 sec. Cool and then add dil. H_2SO_4.	blue colour	
2. Test for Sulphur (S)		
(a) 1 ml of sodium fusion extract + Acidify with dil. CH_3COOH + 1-2 drops of lead acetate soln.	Black ppt.	'S' is present
(b) 1 ml of sodium fusion extract +1-2 drops of freshly prepared solution of sodium nitroprusside solution + dil. NaOH soln.	A deep red or purple colouration	'S' is present
3. Test for Halogens (X)		
(a) 1-2 ml of sodium fusion extract + 2-3 drops of dil. HNO_3 boil and cool + 2 ml of $AgNO_3$.	White or yellow ppt.	'Cl' present
(b) 1 ml of sodium fusion extract + dil. HNO_3 + 2 ml CCl_4 +2 ml chlorine water. Shake the contents	Brown colouration is observed in CCl_4 layer	'Br' present
	Violet colour of CCl_4 layer indicates	'I' present
Test for Nitrogen and Sulphur when present together		
(a) Sodium fusion extract + dil. HCl (3-4 drops) + (1-2 drops) $FeCl_3$ solution.	Blood red colouration	'N' and 'S' present

Test	Observation	Inference
(b) 1 ml of sodium fusion extract + 1 ml of dil. HCl + 2 ml of alcohol + (2-3 drops of cobalt nitrate).	Blue colour	'N' and 'S' present

CHAPTER

2

Test for Functional Groups

Test	*Observation*	*Inference*
(A) TEST FOR CARBOXYLIC ACID (—COOH)		
1. Shake a small amount of O.C.* with water + Dip a blue litmus paper.	Turns red	Carboxylic group present (Phenol being acidic in nature also give this test)
2. Add a pinch of the given O.C. (or a few drops, if liquid) to 5 ml of 50% $NaHCO_3$ solution, and shake gently.	O.C. dissolves with effer-vescences of CO_2	Carboxylic group present (Phenols are mostly insoluble in $NaHCO_3$ soln.
3. 0.2g of O.C. (or 0.5 ml, if liquid) + 1 ml of ethanol + 2-3 drops of conc. H_2SO_4. Heat on a water bath.	Pleasant smell of ester	Carboxylic group present

*O.C.: Organic Compound.

Test	*Observation*	*Inference*
(B) TEST FOR PHENOLS		
1. O.C. + 5% NaOH	O.C. dissolves and reappears by conc. HCl	Phenolic group present
2. Libermann's Test 0.2 g of O.C. + few crystals of $NaNO_2$ in a dry test tube Heat and Cool + 1 ml of conc. H_2SO_4 and shake.	Deep green or blue colour ↓ Add excess dist. water Red ↓ Add excess NaOH soln. Deep green or blue	Phenolic group present
3. $FeCl_3$ Test 1 ml (or 0.2 g) of aq. or alc. solution of O.C. + 2-3 drops of neutral or very dilute soln. of $FeCl_3$.	Blue, red violet colouration	Phenolic group present
4. Phthalein Test 0.2 g of organic compound in a dry test tube + 1 ml phthalic anhydride + 0.5 ml conc. H_2SO_4.	Red colour	Phenol, O-cresol
Heat and Cool, then add to a beaker containing very dilute NaOH solution.	Red solution with green fluorescence	Resorcinol
	Blue colour	Catechol m-cresol
	Green fluorescence	α-Naphthol

Test	*Observation*	*Inference*
5. Azo Dye Test		
0.5 ml aniline + conc. HCl. Cool to 0-5°C + $NaNO_2$ in water + O.C. in NaOH.	Red azo dye	Phenolic group present

* **Preparation of Neutral $FeCl_3$:** Add dil. NH_4OH solution drop by drop in $FeCl_3$ solution until ppt. are formed. Filter it and use the filtrate for the test.

TEST FOR ALCOHOLS (—OH)

Test	Observation	Inference
1. In a dry test tube, take 2 ml of O.C. + a small piece of sodium metal.	Sodium dissolves with evolution of H_2	Alcoholic group present
2. 0.2 g (or 0.5 ml of liquid) of O.C. + 3-4 drops of glacial CH_3COOH + 3-4 drops of conc. H_2SO_4. Heat on a water bath.	Fruity smell of ester	Alcoholic group present
3. 0.2 gm of O.C. in 1 ml of water (or dioxane for water insoluble compounds) + 1 ml ceric ammonium nitrate solution.	Red colour If green brown colour is obtained	Alcoholic group present Phenolic group
4. **Xanthate Test** 0.5 ml of O.C. + a pallet of KOH warm it till the pallet dissolve. Cool + 5-6 drops of CS_2 and shake.	Yellow ppt.	Alcoholic group present. This test is +ve for primary, secondary and tertiary alcohols

Test	Observation	Inference
Distinction between Primary, Sec. and Tert. Alcohols		
2 ml of Lucas reagent (anhy. $ZnCl_2$ + conc. HC1) + 3-4 drops of O.C.	Immediate separation of two phases	Tertiary alcohol
Shake the mixture and wait for 5 minutes.	Cloudy in 2-5 minutes	Secondary alcohol
	Solution remains clear	Primary alcohol

(C) TEST FOR CARBONYL GROUP

0.2 g of O.C. in alcohol + 2, 4-dinitrophenyl-hydrazine (2, 4-DNP).	Bright orange solid separates out	Carbonyl group present

Preparation of Tollen's Reagent

5 ml of $AgNO_3$ solution + 1 ml of 10% NaOH solution and shake. A white ppt. is obtained + NH_4OH solution drop by drop till the ppt. just dissolves.

(D) TEST FOR ALDEHYDE (—CHO GROUP)

1. Tollen's Test		
0.2 g (or 0.5 ml if liquid) of O.C. + Tollen's reagent. Heat.	Metallic Ag-mirror or greyish black ppts	Aldehyde group present
2. Schiffs Test		
1 ml of Schiffs reagent + 4-5 drops of unknown O.C. shake well.	Red or purple colouration	Aldehyde group present
3. Test with Fehling's Solution		
1 ml of O.C. + 5 ml of Fehling's solution	Red ppt. (Benzaldehyde	Aldehyde group

Test	*Observation*	*Inference*
(equal volumes of Fehling's soln. A and Fehling's soln. B) Heat to boiling.	does not reduce Fehling's solution so does not give this test)	present

4. Benedict's Test : Given by only aliphatic aldehydes.

4 ml of Benedict's reagent + 3-4 drops of unknown O.C. (if solid then dissolve it	Red ppt. or	Aliphatic aldehyde
in ethanol or water). Heat to boiling.	Brown colour	Reducing sugar

(This test distinguishes between aliphatic and aromatic aldehyde.)

Ketones respond negatively to the above tests and thus can be distinguished from aldehyde.

(E) TEST FOR KETONE (—C=O) GROUP

1. Iodoform Test : Given by ketones containing $-\overset{\overset{\displaystyle O}{\|}}{C}-CH_3$ group.

0.2 g (0.5 ml of liquid) of unknown O.C. in 2 ml of water (or dioxane or methanol) +1 ml of 10% NaOH solution + Iodine-KI reagent dropwise until a permanent dark colour of iodine persists + 5-7 ml of water. Wait for 15 minutes.	Yellow ppt. of iodoform (m.p. 120°C)	This test is given by aliphatic ketones, mixed ketones and alcohols

2. m-Dinitrobenzene Test

0.2 g unknown O.C. in ethanol + 1% m-dinitrobenzene in ethanol + 2 drops of NaOH solution.	Red colour develops immediately	Acetone/ methyl ethyl ketone/ acetohenone

Test	Observation	Inference
	Light red colour deepens on standing	Benzophenone, Benzaldehyde
	Yellow colour turns pink on standing	Salicylaldehyde
3. 0.5 ml unknown O.C. + saturated sodium bisulphite ($NaHSO_3$) solution and shake vigrously, warm and cool.	White ppt. on cooling (Acetophenone does not respond to this test)	Ketone group present
4. 0.5 ml unknown O.C. + sodium nitroprusside solution + dil. NaOH.	Pink or red or violet colour	Ketone group present

(F) TEST FOR ESTER (—COOR) GROUP

1. Phenolphthalein Test		
2 drops of NaOH solution in test tube + Half test tube distilled water + 2 drops of phenolphthalein (Pink colour appears) + 0.5 ml of unknown O.C. in 2 ml of ethanol. Heat.	Disappearance of pink colour	Ester present
2. Hydroxamic Acid Test		
1 ml unknown O.C. + 0.1 g Hydroxylamine hydrochloride in ethanol + 5 ml of 10% NaOH solution. Boil for 1 to 2 minutes. Cool and acidify with dil. HC1 + 1-2 drops of $FeCl_3$ soln.	Red violet or deep red colouration	Ester present

Test	*Observation*	*Inference*

(G) TEST FOR NITRO GROUP

Test	Observation	Inference
1. Mulliken Barker Test 0.2 g of unknown O.C. in 2 ml ethanol + 3-4 drops of $CaCl_2$ solution + A pinch of Zn dust. Boil, cool and filter in Tollen's reagent.	Black ppts.	Nitro group present
2. 0.2 gm of unknown O.C. + 2 ml of 5% ferrous ammonium sulphate + 1 drop of dil. H_2SO_4 followed by 1 ml of KOH solution in methanol. Shake vigorously.	Red brown ppt.	Nitro group present
3. 0.2 g of unknown O.C. + 2 ml of conc. HC1. + 1 g solid $SnCl_2$ or tin granules. Heat to boiling and perform the primary amine test (Dye test).		

(H) TEST FOR AMINES

Amines are insoluble in water but soluble in mineral acids.

1. Diazotization Test

Test tube No. 1 :
0.2 g of unknown O.C. + 2 ml of dil HC1. Cool to 0-5°C.

Test tube No. 2 :
1 ml of 10% aq. $NaNO_2$ solution. Cool to 0-5°C.

Test	Observation	Inference
Test tube No. 3 : 0.1 g of β-naphthol in 2 ml of 10% NaOH solution. Cool to 0-5°C. Mix test tube no. 1 and test tube no. 2 with shaking followed by test tube No. 3.	Orange to Red azo dye	Primary aryl amine present
2. Carbylamine Test,***		
Dissolve 0.2 g of unknown O.C. in alcoholic NaOH solution + 3-4 drops of chloroform. Warm gently.	Foul odour of isocyanide	Primary amine present (Both aliphatic and aromatic amine give this test)
3. 0.2 g of unknown O.C. + 1 ml dil. HCl + 1 ml of 10% $NaNO_2$ solution in water + 2 ml of 10% NaOH solution.	Yellow solid or oily liquid separates	Secondary amine present
	Dark green oil or solid separates out	Tertiary amine present

(I) TEST FOR AMIDE (—$CONH_2$) GROUP

Test	Observation	Inference
1. 0.2 g of unknown O.C. + 1 ml of 10% NaOH solution. Boil.	Smell of ammonia or white fumes with glass rod dipped in HCl	Amide group present

Note : This test fails if hydrogen at the nitrogen atom is replaced by an alkyl or aryl group.

** This test is negative for sec. and tert. amines.

* After carbylamine test, the mixture should be acidified with HCl and then pour into the sink, or waste container.

Test	*Observation*	*Inference*
2. Hydroxamic Acid Test		
0.2 g of unknown O.C. + 0.2 g of hydroxylamine hydro-chloride + 5 ml of 10% NaOH solution. Boil for 2-3 minutes. Cool + 3-4 drops of $FeCl_3$ soln.	Red colouration	Amide group present

The following tests of Urea may be noted.

3. Biuret Test		
0.2 g of urea (or unknown O.C. in a dry test tube. Heat until the melted organic compound just solidifies. Dissolve the solid in 1 ml of 10% NaOH solution. Cool + 1-2 drops of very dilute copper sulphate solution.	Violet or Purple colouration	Urea present
4. Urea Nitrate Test		
0.2 g of urea in 2 ml of distilled water + 2 ml of conc. HNO_3 cool.	White crystalline ppt. of urea nitrate m.p. 163°C	Urea present

(J) TEST FOR ANILIDE (NHCOR) GROUP

1. Tafel's Test		
0.2 g of unknown O.C. + 5 ml of conc. H_2SO_4 shake. + 0.2 g of $K_2Cr_2O_7$	Red or Violet colour, which changes to green on standing	Anilide present

Test	Observation	Inference
2. Hydrolysis Test		
0.2 g of unknown organic compound + 5 ml dil. HCl. Boil and cool to 0-5°C + $NaNO_2$ in water + β-Naphthol in NaOH.	Red azo dye	Anilide present

(K) TEST FOR HYDROCARBONS

Test	Observation	Inference
1. 0.2 g of unknown O.C. + conc. H_2SO_4 and solid $K_2Cr_2O_7$ and shake.	Green colour	Hydro-carbon present

(L) TEST FOR CARBOHYDRATES

Test	Observation	Inference
1. Blackening with H_2SO_4 0.2 g of unknown O.C. + 1 ml of conc. H_2SO_4	Charring takes place	Carbo-hydrates present
2. Molisch's Test		
Dissolve 0.2 gm of unknown O.C. in 1 ml of water + 3-4 drops of 10% solution of α-naphthol in ethanol + 1-2 ml of conc. H_2SO_4 from the side of the test tube.	A reddish violet ring at the junction of the two liquids.	Carbo-hydrate present glucose fructose, sucrose lactose and maltose give this test
3. Benedict's Test		
Dissolve 0.2 g of unknown O.C. in 2 ml of water + 2 ml of Benedict's reagent. Boil and cool	Red ppt. Solution remains clear	Reducing sugar Non-reduc-ing sugar
4. Barfoed's Test (Test for Monosaccharides)		
Dissolve 0.2 g of unknown O.C. in 2 ml of water + 1 ml of oxide Barfoed's reagent. Heat on water bath.	Red ppt. of cuperous	Indicates Mono-sacchar-ides

Test	Observation	Inference

5. Rapid Furfural Test

0.2 g carbohydrates in 2 ml water + 2-3 drops of 10% solution of α-naphthol in ethanol + 5 ml conc. HCl from the side of the test tube and then boil.

Violet colouration is produced at different rates according to the carbohydrates used.

Fructose Sucrose	Violet colour produced immediately when solution starts to boil.
Glucose Maltose Lactose	Colouration is delayed and produced only after 1 min. of boiling.

In this way glucose may be distinguished from fructose.

6. Action of 10% NaOH Soln.

Boil 0.2 g glucose + 5 ml 10% NaOH.

↓

Mixture turns yellow, and finally brown and emits odour of caramel.

Fructose, Maltose, lactose and soluble starch behave similarly.

Sucrose and ordinary starch do not give colouration.

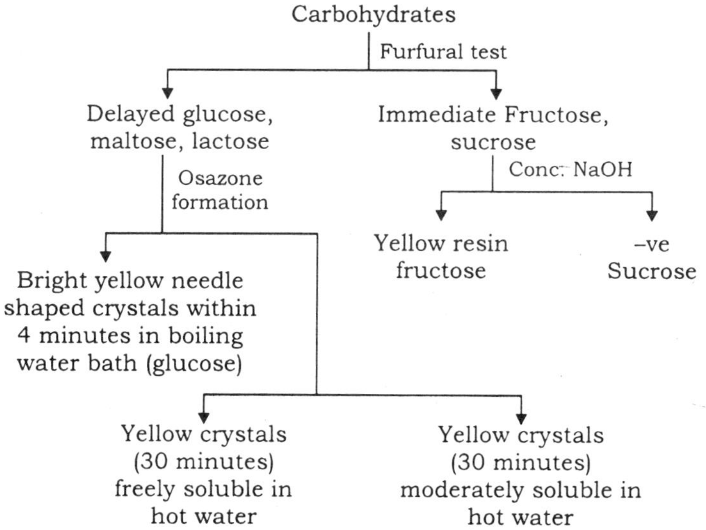

Test	*Observation*	*Inference*

(M) TEST FOR THIOUREA (when N and S present together)

Test	Observation	Inference
1. 0.2 g of unknown O.C. (thiourea) + 2 ml of 10% NaOH soln. Heat.	Smell of ammonia	Thiourea may be present
2. 0.2 g of unknown O.C. + 1 ml of 5% NaOH. Heat, Cool + Lead acetate.	Brown or black ppt.	Thiourea present
3. Dissolve 0.2 g of unknown O.C. in 2 ml of dil. CH_3COOH. Heat + 2 ml of $K_4[Fe(CN)_6]$ solution.	Green colour turns blue on heating	Thiourea present

CHAPTER

3

Melting and Boiling Point Determinations

Melting Point Determination : The melting point of a compound is the constant temperature at which the solid and liquid phase are in equilibrium at one atmospheric pressure.

Determination of Melting Point

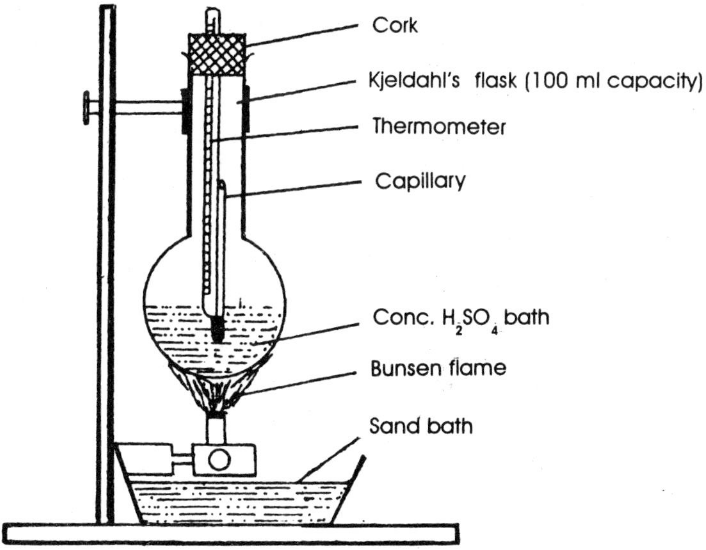

Fig. 3.1: Determination of Melting Point

1. Powder the (crystalline) compound whose m.p. is to be determined on a porous plate with the help of a spatula.
2. Take a capillary tube (about 5 cm) and seal one end by heating it in a bunsen flame.
3. Fill the powdered compound in this capillary tube to a height of about 0.5 cm or 1 cm.
4. Dip 6 cm lower portion of the thermometer (from the mercury side) in the conc. H_2SO_4 bath.
5. Take it out from the acid bath and attach a filled capillary tube with its sealed end near the bulb of thermometer (due to the surface tension and viscosity of the conc. H_2SO_4 bath, the capillary clings to the thermometer).
6. Insert thermometer, with the tube attached, into the centre of the bath slowly. Open end of the capillary should be outside the liquid.
7. At the neck of the Kjeldahl's flask, fix up a thermometer through a cork, having a shallow vertical groove cut or filled to allow expansion of the contents of the Kjeldahl's flask.
8. Heat the flask slowly and rotate the flame over the flask so that the temp. of the bath rises uniformly.
9. As the organic compound in the capillary starts melting, remove the burner at once. The temperature will now rise very slowly.
10. Note the temperature at which the substance begins to liquify and the temperature at which the liquid is clear. Record this interval of temperature as the melting point range of the substance.

Boiling Point Determination: The boiling point of a liquid is that temperature, at which the vapour pressure of a liquid is equal to the atmospheric pressure, the liquid boils freely at this temperature.

Determination of Boiling Point

Method I : As shown in Fig. 3.2 the liquid whose boiling point is to be determined is taken in a distillation flask

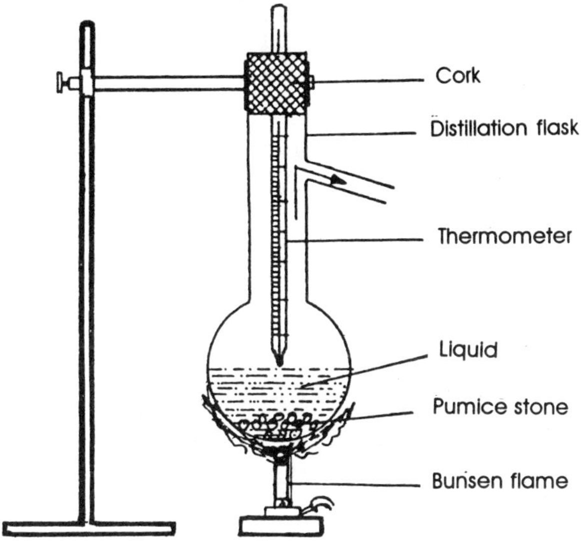

Fig. 3.2: Determination of Boiling Point

(or a test tube like flask with an outlet at the top from where the vapours are collected in a tube). Some pumice stone or porcelain pieces are added to avoid bumping. A thermometer fitted in the flask is connected to a water condenser. If the condenser is not provided, vapours can be collected in a test tube also.

Heat the flask slowly and rise in temperature is carefully observed. The liquid begins to distil over after some time. The bulk of the liquid distils over within a certain temperature range, which remains constant throughout the distillation. This temperature range is taken to be the boiling point of the liquid. This method is useful in the sense, that in addition to determine the boiling point, one is able to purify the given liquid by distillation.

Method II : Siwolowoff's Method for the Determination of the Boiling Point

This method is used when only minute quantities of liquid are available. In an ignition tube take 0.5 ml of

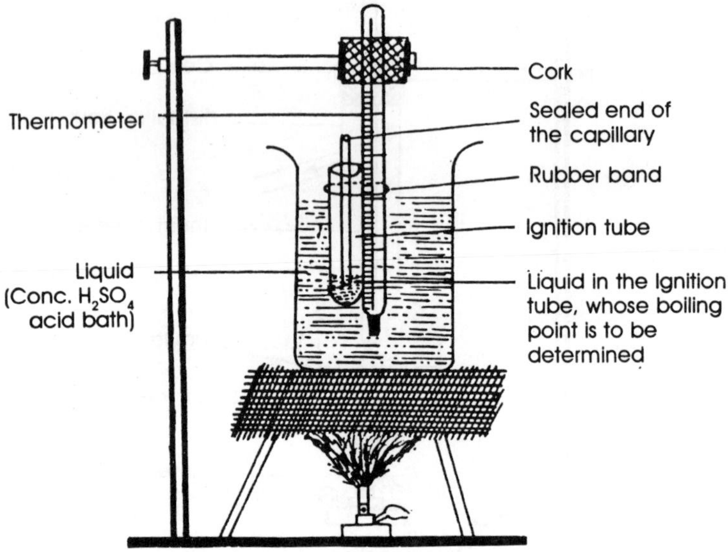

Fig. 3.3: Siwolowoff's Method

the liquid, whose boiling point is to be determined and drop a capillary tube (sealed at the upper end) in it. Attach the ignition tube containing the liquid and the capillary with a thermometer by means of rubber band. Fix the thermometer carrying the ignition tube in a beaker or boiling tube containing conc. H_2SO_4 bath as shown in Fig. 3.3. Heat the beaker with the help of a small rotating flame. Bubbles of air trapped in the inverted capillary will force their way out as the temperature rises. At first a bubble or two will be seen escaping at the end of the capillary dipping in the liquid. The frequency of the bubbles will increase as the boiling point is reached. As soon as a regular stream of bubbles escapes from the capillary, note the temperature at once. It is the boiling point of the liquid.

Determination of Mixed Melting Point

The presence of impurities causes deviation in the melting point. The mixed melting point, therefore, is determined to establish the purity of the substance. In this technique the compound under investigation is mixed with a little amount of same pure compound. The mixture so obtained is filled in the capillary and the melting point determined in the usual manner. If the value of the m.p. of the mixture is lower than that of pure compound then the compound under investigation is impure. If the m.p. of the mixture is same as that of pure compound then the compound under investigation is pure. Sometimes, the deviation in the mixed melting point may be due to the formation of an additional compound on mixing the components. Thus, identification by mixed melting point is although a valuable and frequently used process yet it suffers from some defects and should be used with reasonable care, i.e. keeping in mind the possibility of the formation of new compound or optical isomers.

CHAPTER

4

Preparation of Derivatives with Melting Points

Choice of a Suitable Derivative

A suitable derivative must fulfill the following requirements:

(a) The derivative should be a solid, melting between 70-250°C.

(b) It should be easily prepared in good yields.

(c) The selected derivative should be one which singles out one compound from all the possibilities.

(d) The reagent used in the preparation of derivatives should be readily available.

(e) The physical and chemical properties of derivatives should be markedly different from those of the original compound.

Preparation of Suitable Derivatives

The following derivatives are usually prepared for different classes of organic compounds :

Class of organic compounds	*Suitable derivatives*
Acids	Amides, anilides, s-Benzylisothiouronium salts

Class of organic compounds	*Suitable derivatives*
Phenols	Benzoates, Bromo, 3, 5-dinitrobenzoates
Alcohols	Acetates, p-Nitrobenzoates, Benzoates.
Aldehydes and Ketones	Phenyl hydrazones, 2, 4-Dinitrophenyl hydrazones, Semicarbazones, oximes.
Esters	Amide, isolation of components acid and alcohol. These components serve as a derivatives.
Amines	Acetyl, Benzoyl, Bromo, 2, 4-Dinitrophenyl,
Picrates	
Amides and Anilides	Nitro, Bromo, Picrates
Nitro	
(a) Nitrohydrocarbon	May be reduced to amino compounds and then characterised.
	May be further nitrated, e.g. nitrobenzene on nitration gives m-Dinitrobenzene.
(b) Nitrophenols	Benzoyl, acetyl.
Hydrocarbons	Nitro, Picrates, Oxidation of side chains.
Carbohydrates	Osazone, Acetate
Sulphonic acids	Sulphonamides, sulphonanilides.

1. DERIVATIVES OF CARBOXYLIC ACIDS

(a) Amides

$$RCOOH + PCl_5 \longrightarrow RCOCl + POCl_3 + HCl$$
$$RCOCl + NH_3 \longrightarrow RCONH_2 + HCl$$

Grind 0.5 g of the carboxylic acid and 2 g PCl_5 until the mixture becomes liquid + 10 ml of conc. NH_4OH (liquor NH_3) Stir, cool, filter the solid product (amide). Wash it with cold water, and crystallize from ethanol.

(b) s-Benzylisothiouronium Salts

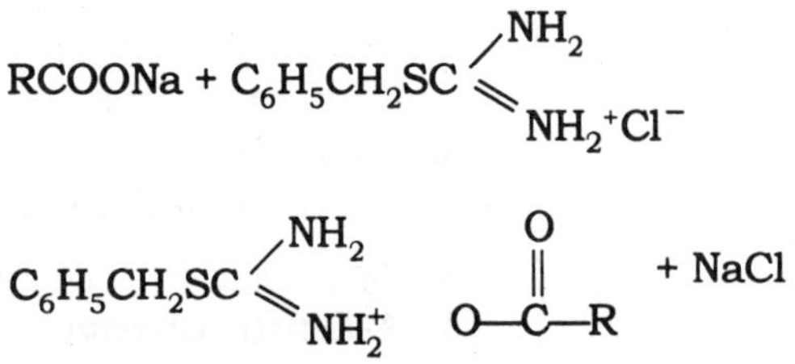

Dissolve 0.5 g of carboxylic acid in 5 ml of distilled water + 2 drops of phenolphthalein + 1N NaOH solution, till a pink colour is obtained + 1 g of s-benzylisothiouronium chloride dissolved in 5 ml of distilled water, cool in ice bath. Filter and recrystallize from aqueous ethanol.

$$ROOH + PCl_5 \longrightarrow RCOCl + POCl_3 + HCl$$
$$ROCl + C_6H_5NH_2 \xrightarrow{NaOH} RCONH + C_6H_5 + HCl$$

(c) Anilides

In a procelain dish take 0.5 g of organic compound + 2 g of PCl_5 + Grind them till it changes to a liquid + 5 ml of acetone. Transfer the contents to a 100 ml flask + 1 ml of aniline and cool + 30 ml of aq NaOH solution. Shake vigorously for fifteen minutes. Filter the solid product obtained. Recrystallize from methanol.

(d) p-Bromo-m-Phenacyl Esters

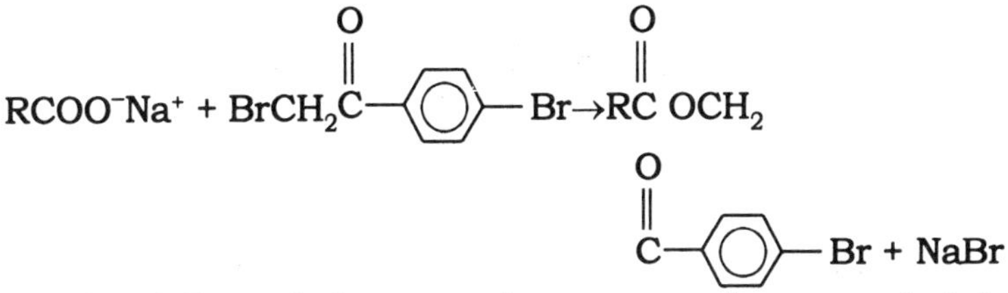

Take 0.5 g of the organic compound suspended in 3 ml of water + 10% NaOH to neutralize the organic compound + 5 ml of ethyl alcohol + 0.5 g of p-Bromophenacyl bromide and reflux for half an hour. Cool and collect the solid. Recrystallize from ethanol.

2. DERIVATIVES OF ALCOHOLS

(a) Acetates

$$ROH + (CH_3CO)_2O \xrightarrow{\text{Pyridine}} RO\overset{\overset{\Large O}{\|}}{C}-CH_3 + CH_3COOH$$

0.5 g (20 drops of liquid) of alcohol + 5 ml pyridine + 3 ml of acetic anhydride with constant shaking. Heat on a water bath for 5 minutes. Pour the contents into ice. Filter, wash with cold water. Recrystallize from aqueous ethanol. (Tertiary alcohols do not give this reaction)

(b) Benzoates

$$C_6H_5COCl + ROH \longrightarrow C_6H_5COOR + HCl$$

1 ml of organic compound + 10 ml acetone + 5 ml benzoyl chloride + 50 ml of aq. NaOH solution. Shake vigorously till the odour of benzoyl chloride disappears. Filter, wash well with water. Recrystallize from alcohol.

(c) p-Nitro Benzoates

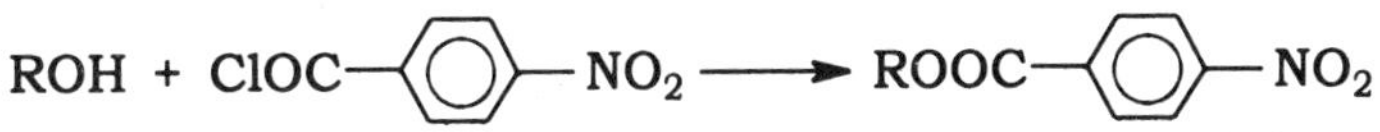

Table 4.1 : Organic acids with suitable derivatives and melting points

Name of the organic compound (Solid acids)	*m.p. °C*		*Solubility*	*Derivatives and their m.p. °C*			
	Aliphatic	*Aromatic*		*Amides*	*Anilides*	*s-Benzoyl isothiouranium salts*	*p-Bromo phenacyl esters*
Phenyl acetic acid		76	Hot water	157	117	165	89
Oxalic acid	101		Sol. in water		245	198	242
o-Toluic acid		102	Sp. sol. in water	143	125	146	–
m-Toluic acid		109	Sp. sol. in water	94	–	–	–
p-Toluic acid		178	Sol. in hot water	158	140	190	153
Benzoic acid		121	Sol. in hot water	129	160	167	119
Cinnamic acid		133	Sp. sol. in water	141	153	–	145
Acetylsalicylic acid		135	Sol. in water	(Salicylic acid - 155)			
o-Chlorobenzoic acid		141	Sol. in hot water	139	114		107
m-Chlorobenzoic acid		158	Sp. sol. in water	134	–	–	–
p-Chlorobenzoic acid		236	Sp. sol. in water	201	194	182	136
o-Bromobenzoic acid		150	Sp. in hot water	155	141	171	–
m-Bromobenzoic acid		155	Sp. sol. in water	155	137	168	126
p-Bromobenzoic acid		251	Sp. sol. in hot water	189	197	–	–

*Sp. = Sparingly

Name of the organic compound (Solid acids)	m.p.°C		Solubility	Derivatives and their m.p.°C			
	Aliphatic	*Aromatic*		*Amides*	*Anilides*	*s-Benzoyl isothiouranium salts*	*p-Bromo phenacyl esters*
o-Bromobenzoic acid		150	Sol. in hot water	155	141	171	–
m-Bromobenzoic acid		155	Sp. sol. in water	155	137	168	126
p-Bromobenzoic acid		251	Sp. sol. in hot water	189	197	–	–
o-Nitrobenzoic acid		147	Sp. in hot water	175	155	109	107
m-Nitrobenzoic acid		140	Sol. in hot water	142	153	–	–
p-Nitrobenzoic acid		241	Sp. sol. in water and alcohol	201	204	–	–
Anthranilic acid (o-Aminobenzoic acid)		146	Sol. in water and alcohol	109	–	149	172
m-Aminobenzoic acid		174	Sol. in hot water and alcohol	75	129	–	–
p-Aminobenzoic acid		188	Sol. in hot water	114	–	–	–
Salicylic acid		158	Sol. in water	139	134	148	140
Adipic acid		152	Sol. in alcohol Sp. sol in water	220	235	163	165
α-Naphthoic acid		160	Sp. sol. in water	202	160	–	–
β-Naphthoic acid		182	Insol. in water	192	170	–	–

Table 4.1

Name of the organic compound (Solid acids)	m.p.°C		Solubility	Derivatives and their m.p.°C			
	Aliphatic	Aromatic		Amides	Anilides	s-Benzoyl isothiouranium salts	p-Bromo phenacyl esters
Anisic acid		184	Sp. sol. in water	162	168		–
Succinic acid	185		Sol. in water	245	226	154	211
Hippuric acid		187	Sol. in hot water and alcohol	–	–	–	–
Phthalic acid		195 (d)**	Sol. in hot water	220	–	158	154
						(Anhydride-130)	
Liquid acids							
Formic acid	101		Miscible with water	–	50	–	–
Acetic acid	118		Miscible with water	82	115	–	–
Propionic acid	141		Miscible with water	–	106	–	–
Isobutyric acid	155		Miscible with water	129	105	–	–
n-Butyric acid	163		Miscible with water	115	96	–	–
Pyruvic acid	165	(d)	Sol. in water	–	–	–	–
				(2,4 dinitro phenyl hydrazone - 213)			
α-Chloro propionic acid	186		Miscible with water	80	92	–	–
Dichloro acetic acid	190		Miscible with water	96	118	–	–

**d–decomposition.

1 ml of organic compounds (4 ml pyridine) + 1 g of p-nitro benenzoyl chloride. Shake well, boil for a few minutes. Pour the mixture into 10 ml of ice water with stirring. Filter, wash with Na_2CO_3 soln. Recrystallize from alcohol.

(Tertiary alcohols do not give this reaction.)

3. DERIVATIVES OF PHENOLS

The derivatives prepared for alcohols can be prepared for phenols also. In addition, the following derivatives may also be prepared.

(a) Benzoates

$$C_6H_5OH + C_6H_5COCl \xrightarrow{\text{Base}} C_6H_5O{-}\overset{\overset{\displaystyle O}{\|}}{C}{-}C_6H_5$$

0.5 ml of phenol + 3 ml water + 3 ml of 10% NaOH soln. + 0.5 ml Benzoyl chloride. Stopper the tube and shake for several minutes, till the odour of benzoyl chloride disappears. Filter wash with cold water. Recrystallize from alcohol.

(b) Acetates

Procedure is same as in case of alcohols.

(c) 3,5-Dinitrobenzoates

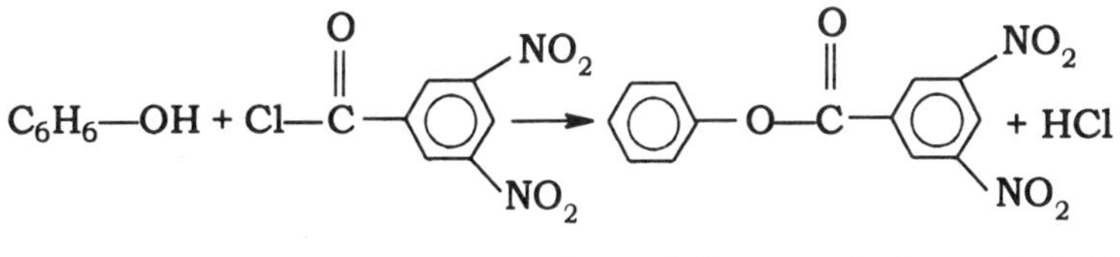

0.5 g of phenol + 5 ml pyridine + 0.5 g of 3,5-dinitrobenzoyl chloride. Reflux for 1 hour, cool and pour into 30 ml of 5% H_2SO_4. Filter, wash with water. Recrystallize from aq. ethanol.

(d) 2,4-Dinitrophenyl Ether

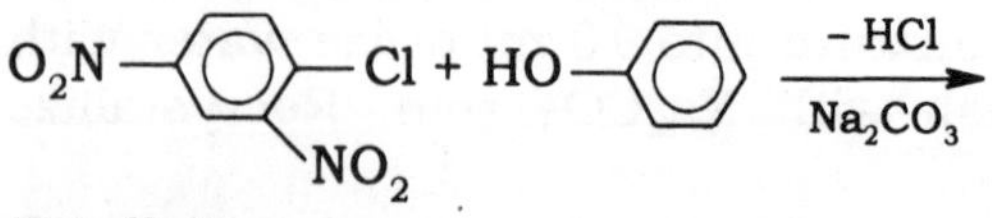

(2,4-dinitro
Chloro benzene)

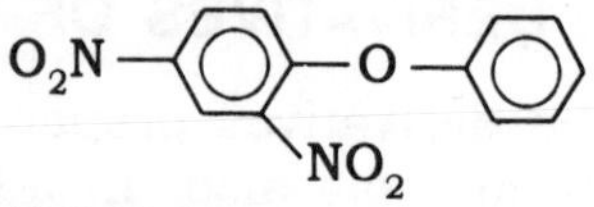

(2,4-dinitro
phenyl ether)

0.5 g phenol + 0.5 g 2,4-dinitrochloro benzene + 5 ml aq. Na_2CO_3 solution + 10 ml alcohol. Reflux by using air condenser for 20 minutes + 20 ml water. Cool, filter it, wash it with water. Recrystallize from alcohol.

(e) Picrates

A few phenols, e.g. α and β-naphthols, etc. form picrates 0.2 g organic compound in 2 ml benzene + 2 ml saturated soln. of picric acid in benzene. Shake till the solid product separates out. Filter, wash with a few drops of benzene. Dry it and determine m.p.

4. DERIVATIVES OF ALDEHYDES AND KETONES

(a) Phenyl Hydrazones

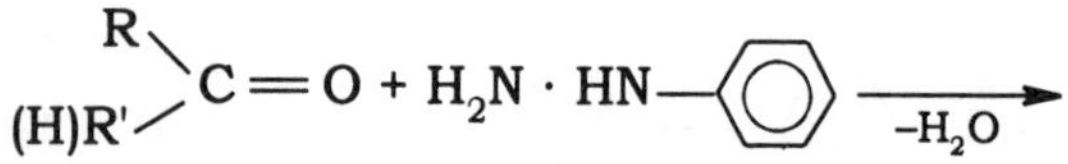

(Phenyl Hydrazine)

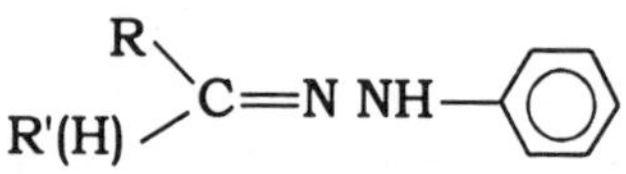

(Phenyl Hydrazone)

Take 0.5 g phenyl hydrazine hydrochloride + 1 g sodium acetate + 5 ml water. Shake the contents to dissolve + 0.5 g of carbonyl compound in 5 ml methanol. Shake and boil on a waterbath for 15 minutes, cool, filter. Recrystallize from aq. ethanol.

(b) 2,4-Dinitrophenyl Hydrazones

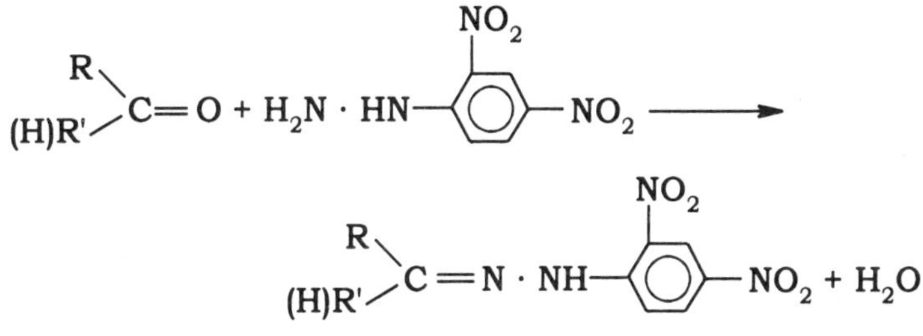

In a dry test tube take 0.2 g of 2, 4-dinitrophenyl hydrazine + 10 ml of methanol + 5 drops of conc. HCl, warm and cool + 0.2 g of aldehyde (or ketone) dissolved in 2 ml of methanol. Warm in a water bath for 15-20 minutes and then allow to stand for 15 minutes at room temperature + water till precipitation is complete. Filter, recrystallize from aq. ethanol.

(c) Semicarbazones

$$\text{R(H)R'C}{=}\text{O} + \text{H}_2\text{NNHCONH}_2 \longrightarrow \text{R(H)R'C}{=}\text{N}\cdot\text{NHCONH}_2 + \text{H}_2\text{O}$$

Take 0.1 g semicarbazide hydrochloride + 0.2 g sodium acetate + 2 ml water + 2 ml ethanol + 0.2 g (0.2 ml) of aldehyde or ketone. Shake for a few minutes, warm it in a water bath at 75-80°C for 15 minutes and cool it. The semicarbazone crystallizes out from cold solution. Recrystallize from aq. ethanol.

(d) Oximes

$$\text{R(H)R'C}{=}\text{O} + \underset{\text{(Hydroxyl amine)}}{\text{H}_2\text{NOH}} \longrightarrow \underset{\text{(Oxime)}}{\text{R(H)R'C}{=}\text{NOH}} + \text{H}_2\text{O}$$

Table 4.2 : Alcohols and Phenols (their derivatives with m.p. °C)

	m.p. °C			*Derivatives and their m.p. °C*			
Name of the organic compound	*Aliphatic*	*Aromatic*	*Solubility*	*3,5-Dinitro benzoate*	*p-nitro benzoate*	*Acetates*	*Benzoates*
o-Nitro benzyl alcohol		74	Sol. in alcohol	–	–	35	94
p-Nitro benzyl alcohol		93	Sol. in hot water	–	–	78	89
d-Sorbitol	110		Sol. in water	–	–	99	129
d-Mannitol	166		Sol. in water	–	–	121	149
Phenol		43	Sol. in water	146	126		69 (Picrate derivative-83)
o-Nitrophenol		45 (B.P. 216)	Sol. in hot water	155	141	41	142
Thymol		50	Sol. in hot water	103	70	–	–
p-Bromo phenol		64	Sol. in NaOH	191	180	–	102
m-Nitro phenol		97	Sol. in hot water and NaOH	159	174	56	95
α-Naphthol		94	Sol. in alcohol and NaOH	217	143		56 (Picrate-89)

Name of the organic compound	m.p. °C		Solubility	Derivatives and their m.p.°C			
	Aliphatic	*Aromatic*		*3,5-Dinitro benzoate*	*p-nitro benzoate*	*Acetates*	*Benzoates*
Catechol		105	Sol. in water	152	169	63	84
p-Nitrophenol		114		186	159	83	142
Resorcinol		110		201	182	–	117
Picric acid		122		–	143	76	(naphthalene picrate-149 α -Benzone Picrate-84)
β-naphthol		123		186	169	70	–
Pyrogallol		133		205	230	161	89
Hydroquinone		170		317	263	123	199
Phloroglucinol		218		–	–	105	173
Liquids							
Methyl alcohol	65			108	96	–	–
Ethyl alcohol	78			93	57	–	–
Isopropyl alcohol	82			123	110	–	–

(Contd.)

Table 4.2

Name of the organic compound	m.p. °C		Solubility	Derivatives and their m.p. °C			
	Aliphatic	Aromatic		3,5-Dinitro benzoate	p-nitro benzoate	Acetates	Benzoates
n-Propyl alcohol	97			75	35	–	–
(isobuty) alcohol	108			87	69	–	–
tert. butyl alcohol	83			142	116	–	–
n-Butyl alcohol	117			64	36	–	–
Cyclohexanol	116			113	50	–	–
Glycol	198			169	140	–	–
Benzyl alcohol		205		113	85	–	–
Glycerol	290(d)			–	188	–	72
α-decomposition							
o-Chloro phenol		176		143	115	–	– (Picrates-181°C)
p-Chloro phenol		217		186	158	–	–
m-Chloro phenol		214		159	99	–	–
o-Bromo phenol		195		–	–	–	–

(Contd.)

Name of the Organic Compound	m.p. °C		Solubility	Derivatives and their m.p. °C			
	Aliphatic	*Aromatic*		*3,5-Dinitro*	*p-nitro*	*Acetates*	*Benzoates*
							(Tribromo-95, 2,4 dinitrophenyl ester-99)
m-Bromo phenol		236		–	–	–	–
p-Bromo phenol		235 (M.P.64)		191	180	–	–
m-Cresol		202		165	90	–	55
o-Cresol		191		138	94	–	–
p-Cresol		202		189	98	–	71

Take 0.5 g hydroxylamine hydrochloride and dissolve in 2 ml of water + 3 ml of 10% NaOH soln. + 0.5 g carbonyl compound. Shake well + 5 ml ethyl alcohol. Heat for 15 minutes by using air condenser, cool in ice and dilute with 10 ml of water. Filter, and recrystallize from ethanol or benzene.

5. DERIVATIVES OF ESTERS

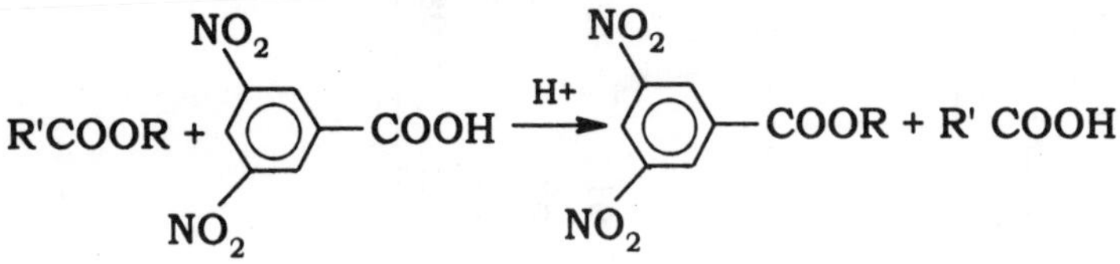

3, 5-dinitrobenzoic acid

Take 0.5 g of ester + 0.5 g 3, 5-dinitrobenzoic acid + 2 drops conc. H_2SO_4. Heat under reflux condition for 10 minutes. Add 10 ml of water, make alkaline with NaOH and filter the solid 3, 5-dinitrobenzoate. Recrystallize from benzene. Determine m.p.

(See the list of alcohols and 3, 5-dinitrobenzoate deriv. list for m.p.)

6. DERIVATIVES OF CARBOHYDRATES

(a) Osazone

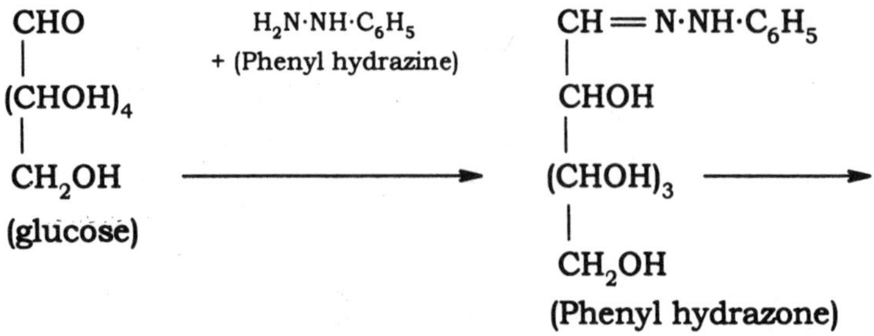

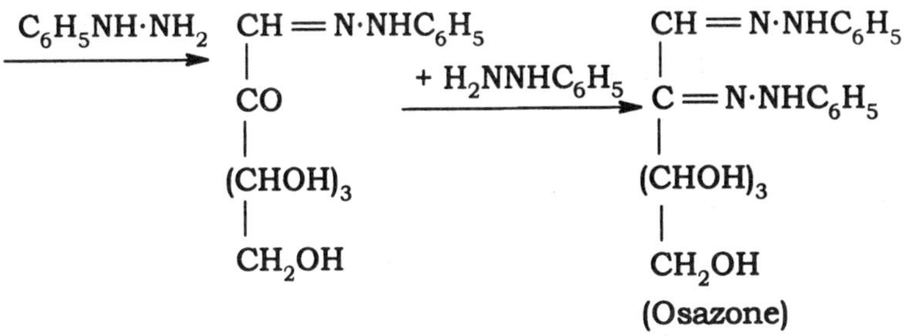

Take 0.5 g of carbohydrate + 1.5 g sodium acetate + 1 g phenyl hydrazine hydrochloride + 10 ml water + 1 ml saturated soln. of sodium bisulphite, stopper the boiling tube loosely with a cork and place it in a boiling water bath. Note the time of osazone formation (precipitation). Osazones of lactose and maltose are soluble in water, which separate on excessive cooling. Melting point of osazones being too close and are of no value.

(b) Oximes

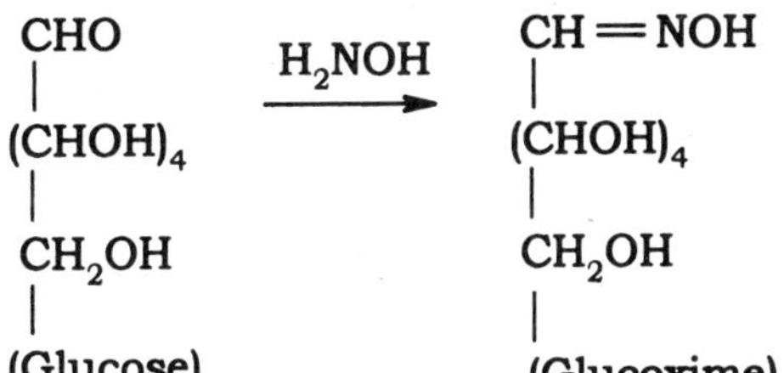

Take 0.5 g hydroxylamine hydrochloride and dissolve in 3 ml of water + 3 ml of 10% NaOH + 0.5 g carbohydrates. Shake + 5 ml ethanol. Heat for 15 minutes by using air condenser. Cool in ice and dilute with 10 ml water, filter, recrystallize from ethanol.

Table 4.3 : Aldehydes and their derivatives

Name of the organic compound	*Aliphatic*		*Aromatic*		*Derivatives and their m.p. °C*		
	m.p.	*b.p.*	*m.p.*	*b.p.*	*Phenyl hydra-zone*	*2,4-dinitro phenyl hydra-zone*	*Semi-carba-zone*
o-Amino benzaldehyde			40		227	250	247
p-Amino benzaldehyde			72		156	194	173
Benzaldehyde				179	158	237	222
o-Bromo benzaldehyde				230	–	–	214
m-Bromo benzaldehyde				234	141	257	205
p-Bromo benzaldehyde			57		113	260	228
Bromal				174	–	–	87
n-Butyraldehyde		74			94	126	95
o-Chloro benzaldehyde					86	207	225
m-Chloro benzaldehyde				213	134	248	228
p-Chloro benzaldehyde			47	214	127	218	230
Crotonaldehyde		104			56	190	201
Chlorol		98			–	131	90(d)
Cinnamaldehyde				247	168	254	215

(Contd.)

Name of the organic compound	Aliphatic		Aromatic		Derivatives and their m.p. °C		
	m.p.	b.p.	m.p.	b.p.	Phenyl hydrazone	2,4-dinitro phenyl hydrazone	Semi-carbazone
Furfural				161	97	229	202
Hexahydro benzaldehyde				162	-	172	173
m-Hydroxy benzaldehyde			104	240	130	260	198
p-Hydroxy benzaldehyde			115	-	177	280	224
o-Methoxy benzaldehyde				243	120	253	215
m-Methoxy benzaldehyde				230	76	219	233
p-Methoxy benzaldehyde				248	120	254	210
Propionaldehyde		49		-	-	155	89
Phenylacetaldehyde				194	58	121	156
Salicylaldehyde				196	142	252	231
o-Tolualdehyde				200	106	193	212
m-Tolualdehyde				199	91	212	216
p-Tolualdehyde				204	121	234	234
Vanillin			80	285	105	271	229
Phthalaldehyde			56	-	191	-	-
o-nitro benzaldehyde			44	252	156	250	256

(Contd.)

Table 4.3

Name of the organic compound	Aliphatic		Aromatic		Derivatives and their m.p. °C		
	m.p.	*b.p.*	*m.p.*	*b.p.*	*Phenyl hydra-zone*	*2,4-dinitro phenyl hydra-zone*	*Semi-carba-zone*
m-nitro benzaldehyde			58	–	120	293	246
p-nitro benzaldehyde			106	–	159	320	221
1-Naphthaldehyde			34	292	80	254	221
2-Naphthaldehyde			60	–	206	270	245
glyoxal		50		–	–	300	270
Formalin		97		–	–	166	169
Anisaldehyde				248	120	254	209

Table 4.4 : Ketones and their derivatives

Name of the organic compound	*Aliphatic*		*Aromatic*		*Derivatives and their m.p. °C*		
	m.p.	*b.p.*	*m.p.*	*b.p.*	*Phenyl hydrazone*	*2,4-dinitro phenyl hydrazone*	*Semicarbazone*
Acetone		56			–	126	190
Acetylacetone		139			273	209	185
Acetonylacetone		194			120	257	224
Acetophenone				202	105	250	198
n-Butyl methyl ketone		128			–	106	122
o-Bromo acetophenone				112	–	189	177
m-Bromo acetophenone				131	–	–	238
p-Bromo acetophenone			51	256	126	230	208
Benzyl methyl ketone			27	216	87	156	198
Benzyl ethyl ketone				226	–	–	135
Benzophenone			49	306	137	239	164
p-Bromo benzophenone			82	350	126	230	–
Benzyl phenyl ketone			60	320	116	204	148
Benzoin			137	344	106	245	206
Benzil			95	347	134	–	182

(contd.)

Table 4.4

Name of the organic compound	Aliphatic		Aromatic		Derivatives and their m.p. °C		
	m.p.	b.p.	m.p.	b.p.	Phenyl hydrazone	2,4-dinitro phenyl hydrazone	Semicarbazone
					(mono) 135 (di-deriv)		(mono) 244 (di-deriv)
Benzalacetone			42	262	157	227	187
Dibenzalacetone			112		153	180	190
Chloroacetone		119			–	125	164
Cyclopentanone		131			55	147	209
Cyclohexanone		156			81	162	166
Cycloheptanone		180			72	148	163
d-Camphor	179	209			233	177	237
o-Chloro acetophenone				229	–	206	160
m-Chloro acetophenone				228	–	–	232
p-Chloro acetophenone				232	114	230	200
p-Chloro benzophenone			78		106	185	–
Diethyl ketone		102			–	156	139
Di-n-propyl ketone		144			–	75	133

(*Contd.*)

Name of the organic compound	Aliphatic		Aromatic		Derivatives and their m.p. °C		
	m.p.	b.p.	m.p.	b.p.	Phenyl hydrazone	2,4-dinitro phenyl hydrazone	Semicarbazone
Di-iso propyl ketone		124			–	88	160
Di-n-butyl ketone		188			–	–	90
Di-p-tolyl ketone			95		100	229	140
Dibenzyl ketone				331	128	100	146
Dibenzalacetone		–	112	–	153	180	190
Ethylmethyl ketone		80		–	–	115	146
Ethyl acetoacetate		181		–	–	93	133
o-Hydroxy acetophenone		–		215	110	–	210
m-Hydroxy acetophenone		–	96	–	–	–	210
p-Hydroxy acetophenone		–	109	–	151	261	199
Isobutyl methyl ketone		117		–	–	95	132
Methyl-n-propyl ketone		102		–	–	144	112
Methyl-isopropyl ketone		94		–	–	120	113
Mesityl oxide		130		–	142	203	133

(Contd.)

Table 4.4

Name of the organic compound	*Aliphatic*		*Aromatic*		*Derivatives and their m.p. °C*		
	m.p.	*b.p.*	*m.p.*	*b.p.*	*Phenyl hydra-zone*	*2,4-dinitro phenyl hydra-zone*	*Semi-carba-zone*
2-Methyl-cyclohexanone		165		–	–	137	197
3-Methyl-cyclohexanone		170	–	–	94	155	190
4-Methyl-cyclohexanone		171	–	–	110	134	198
Methyl-1-naphthyl ketone		–	–	302	146	–	230
Methyl-2-naphthyl ketone		–	–	301	177	262	236
o-Nitroacetophenone		–		218	–	–	–
m-Nitroacetophenone		–	81	–	128	228	257
p-Nitroacetophenone		–	81	–	132	–	–
Pinacolone		106	–	–	–	125	157
Propiophenone		218	147	191	181	–	–
Phenacyl chloride		–	59	–	–	212	156
Phenacyl bromide		–	–	50	–	230	146

(c) Acetates

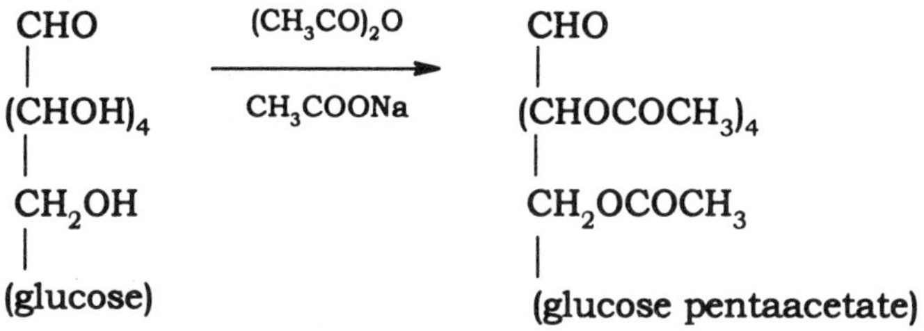

Take 0.5 g carbohydrate + 0.5 g fused sodium acetate + 5 ml acetic anhydride in a dry test tube. Shake, heat for 1 hour using air condenser. Pour reaction mixture into crushed ice. Filter, wash with cold water and recrystallize from ethanol.

(d) Benzoates

Glucose and fructose give crystalline benzoate derivatives. Take 0.5 g glucose + 5 ml water + 10 ml of 15% NaOH solution + 1 ml benzoyl chloride, stopper the boiling tube and shake. Filter the solid. Recrystallize from ethanol.

Compound	*Time of osazone formation*	*Shape of the crystals*
Glucose	4 min.	Bright yellow crystalline needles arranged in fan shaped aggregates.
Fructose	2 min.	Same as in case of glucosazone.
Maltose	30 min. (soluble in hot water)	Yellow crystals arranged in the form of sun flower.
Lactose	30 min. (moderately soluble in hot water)	Yellow crystals arranged in the form of balls of prickles.
Sucrose	30 min.	
Galactose	15 min.	

7. DERIVATIVES OF NITRO COMPOUNDS*

(a) Reduction to Amino Derivatives

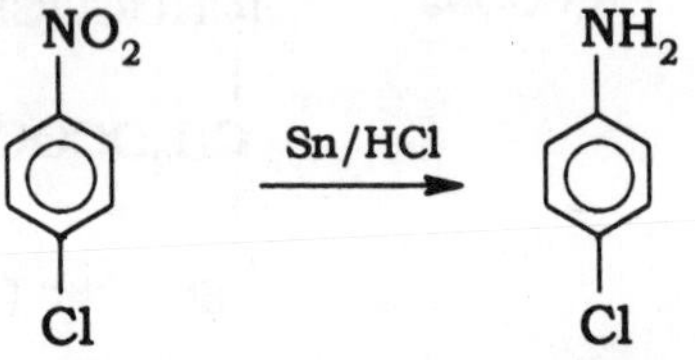

(p-Chloro nitro benzene) (p-Chloro aniline)

1 g of nitro compound + 5 ml ethanol + 2 g granulated tin with constant stirring + 20 ml dil. HCl in small portions with vigrous shaking. Warm on a boiling water bath for 20 minutes + 30 ml of 40% NaOH, extract the soln. with 5 ml portions of ether five to six times. Distlll off ether. Determine.

m.p./b.p. (°C) — The residue is either (a) Aniline (from nitro benzene) p-toluidine (from p-nitrotoluene) or m-phenylene diamine $C_6H_4(NH_2)_2$ (from m-dinitro benzene)

(I) DERIVATIVES OF NITRO-PHENOLS

(a) Benzoyl Derivatives

Take 1 g of nitro-phenols in a boiling tube + 5 ml conc. HCl + 1 g granulated tin with constant stirring. Warm on a boiling water bath for 20 minutes, cool and add 30 ml of 40% NaOH + 10-15 ml benzoyl chloride and shake for five minutes. The dibenzoyl derivative will separate out. Filter, recrystallize from ethanol.

---

* In general, nitro hydrocarbons are readily identified by reduction to the corresponding amines, which is then identified as its benzoyl, acetyl or picrate derivative (Procedure for benzoyl, acetyl or picrate derivative is same as for primary amines).

(b) Acetyl Derivative

Take 1 g nitro phenol + 3 ml acetic anhydride + 5 drops conc. H_2SO_4. Reflux for 15 minutes. Pour into 30 ml water. Solid acetate separate out. Filter, recrystallize from ethanol.

For m.p. see table of primary amines (acetyl and benzoyl derivatives).

(II) DERIVATIVES OF NITRO-ANILINES

Prepare acetyl or benzoyl derivatives as in (1) above For m.p. see table of primary amines (acetyl and benzoyl derivatives).

8. DERIVATIVES OF AMINES

(a) Acetyl Derivative

Take 1 g (or 1 ml) of organic compound + 5 ml acetic anhydride. Reflux for 10 minutes. Pour the reaction mixture into 30 ml water. Filter, wash with cold water. Recrystallize from ethanol.

$$RNH_2 + (CH_3CO)_2O \longrightarrow RNH{\cdot}CO{\cdot}CH_3$$

Primary and secondary amines undergo acetylation.

(b) Benzoyl Derivatives

$$C_6H_5\ COCl + RNH_2 \longrightarrow \underset{\text{(Benzoyl derivative)}}{C_6H_5\ CONHR} + HCl$$

Take 1 ml (or 1 g) of organic compound in a test tube + 20 ml of 10% NaOH soln. + 2 ml benzoyl chloride. Shake vigorously for 10 minutes. Filter it, wash with water. Recrystallize from alcohol.

Primary and secondary amines can undergo benzoylation easily.

(c) Picrate Derivatives

$$R{-}NH_2 + C_6H_2\ (NO_2)_3\ OH \longrightarrow \underset{\text{(Picrate)}}{RNH_2\ C_6H_2\ (NO_2)_3\ OH}$$

Table 4.5 : Carbohydrates and their derivatives m.p. (°C)

Name	*Phenyl osazone*	*Derivatives m.p. (°C)*		
		Oxime derivatives	*Acetate derivative*	
Glucose	205 (formed in 4 min.)	137	Penta-acetate	111
Fructose	205 (formed in 2 min.)	118	–	
Maltose	205 (formed in 30 min.)	–	Octa-acetate	158
Galactose	201 (formed in 15 min.)	175	Penta-acetate	142
Sucrose	205 (formed in 30 min.)	–	Octa-acetate	69
Lactose	200 (formed in 30 min.)	–	Octa-acetate	(95-100)

Table 4.6 : Nitro-compounds

Name of the organic compound	*Aromatic*	
	m.p. (°C)	*b.p. (°C)*
Nitrobenzene		210
m-Dinitrobenzene	90	
o-Nitro-toluene		220
p-Nitro-toluene	52	238
o-Nitro phenol	46	216
m-Nitro phenol	97	
p-Nitro phenol	114	
o-Nitro-aniline	71	
m-Nitro-aniline	114	
p-Nitro-aniline	148	
o-Nitro-benzyl alcohol	74	
p-Nitro-benzyl alcohol	93	
o-Nitro-benzyl chloride	48	
m-Nitro-benzyl chloride	45	
p-Nitro-benzyl chloride	71	
p-Nitro-benzyl bromide	99	
p-Nitro-benzyl iodide	127	
o-Nitro-benzoic acid	148	
m-Nitro-benzoic acid	141	
p-Nitro-benzoic acid	241	
1-Nitro-naphthalene	61	
2-Nitro-naphthalene	79	

Take 0.5 g (0.5 ml) organic compound in 5 ml alcohol + 5 ml of saturated soln. of picric acid in alcohol. Warm the mixture on a water bath for 10 minutes. Cool, filter and recrystallize it from benzene. Picrates are employed as derivatives of tertiary amine.

9. DERIVATIVES OF HYDROCARBONS

(a) Picrates

$$C_{10}H_8 + C_6H_2(NO_2)_3OH \xrightarrow{\text{Benzene}} \underset{\text{(Picrate)}}{C_{10}H_8 \cdot C_6H_2(NO_2)_3OH}$$

Dissolve 0.5 hydrocarbon in hot benzene or hot rectified spirit + 0.5 g picric acid dissolve in hot benzene or hot rectified spirit. Shake, cool and filter Recrystallize from benzene.

(b) Nitroderivatives

(i) **Mono nitration product :** 0.5 g hydrocarbon + 5 ml conc. H_2SO_4 + 2 ml of conc. HNO_3 dropwise. Heat on a water bath at 60-70°C for 15 minutes. Cool and pour reaction mixture on crushed ice. Filter it. Recrystallize from methanol.

(ii) **Dinitration product :** For dinitration product use 6 ml of fuming nitric acid in place of conc. HNO_3. Procedure is same as for mono-nitration.
If excess amount of brown fumes are evolved during nitration, then reaction mixture should be cooled in cold water bath.

(iii) For trinitration product (if possible), add 8 ml of fuming nitric acid. Procedure is same as for mono-nitration.

BROMO DERIVATIVES

Dissolve 1 g (or 1 ml) of organic compound in CCl_4 + 2-3 crystals of I_2 + 2 ml liquid Br_2 dissolved in 5 ml CCl_4. Shake and wait for 5 minutes.

Evaporate CCl_4 from the above mixture on a water bath + 20 ml of hot 5% NaOH to remove I_2 + 10 ml water. Filter the solid, recrystallize from alcohol.

10. DERIVATIVES OF SULPHONIC ACIDS

(a) Sulphonamides (Amides) Derivative

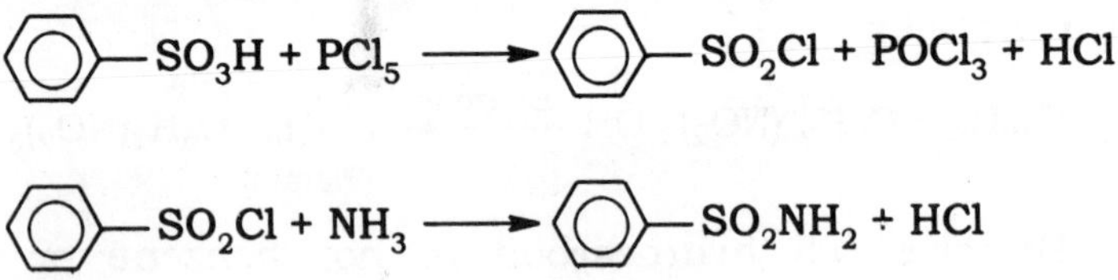

(Benzene sulphonyl chloride) (Benzene sulphonamide)

Take 1 g of organic compound + 3 g of PCl_5 in a 100 ml dry conical flask. Reflux for half an hour. Cool, add 30 ml benzene in the above mixture, warm on a water bath. Shake, filter + 10 ml conc. NH_3 (liquor NH_3) with constant stirring. Evaporate benzene on a water bath. Recrystallize from alcohol.

(b) Sulphonanilides (Anilides) Derivative

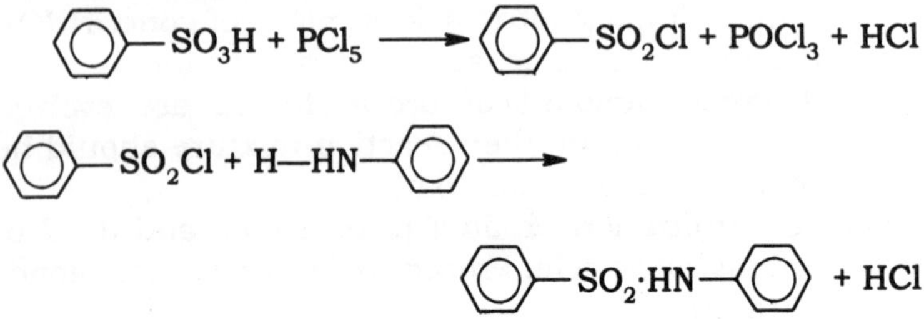

(Sulphonanilide)

Take 1 g of given organic compound in a 100 ml dry conical flask + 3 g PCl_5 + reflux for half an hour. Cool, add 20 ml benzene. Shake, warm + 3 ml (3g) aniline + Heat for half an hour. Cool in an ice bath. Filter the solid product recrystallize from alcohol.

Table 4.7 : Primary Amines and their Derivatives

Name of the organic compound	*Aliphatic*		*Aromatic*		*Derivatives m.p. °C*		
	m.p.	*b.p.*	*m.p.*	*b.p.*	*Picrate*	*Acetyl deriv.*	*Benzoyl deriv.*
Allylamine		56			140	215	–
n-Amylamine		105			143	–	–
Aniline				184	189	114	163
o-Anisidine				225	200	88	60
m-Anisidine				251	169	81	112
p-Anisidine			57	246	165	130	153
o-Aminohenol			174		–	124	184
m-Aminophenol			123		–	101	143
p-Aminophenol			186		–	151	234
p-Amino-dimethyl-aniline			41	262	188	132	228
p-Amino-diethyl-aniline				261	–	104	172
2-Amino-biphenyl			50	300	–	121	102
4-Amino-biphenyl			53	302	–	171	230
n-Butyl amine		77			151	230	70
Benzyl amine				185	199	60	105
o-Bromoaniline				229	129	99	116

(contd.)

Table 4.7

Name of the organic compound	Aliphatic		Aromatic		Derivatives m.p. °C		
	m.p.	b.p.	m.p.	b.p.	Picrate	Acetyl deriv.	Benzoyl deriv.
m-Bromo aniline				251	180	87	120
p-Bromo aniline			66		180	167	204
Benzidine			127	–		317	352
o-Chloroaniline				209	134	88	99
m-Chloroaniline				230	177	79	122
p-chloroaniline			71	232	178	179	192
2,4-Dichloroaniline			63		106	146	117
2,4-Dibromoaniline			79		124	146	134
2,4,6-Trichloro aniline			78		83	206	174
2,4,6-Tribromo aniline			120		–	238	198
4,4'-Diamino biphenyl (Benzidine)			127		–	317	352
Ethylenediamine				117	234	172	249
Iso butylamine		69			156	227	57
o-Iodo-aniline			60		112	110	139
p-Iodo-aniline			64		–	184	222
o-Nitroaniline			72		73	94	98

(contd.)

Name of the organic compound	*Aliphatic*		*Aromatic*		*Derivatives m.p. °C*		
	m.p.	*b.p.*	*m.p.*	*b.p.*	*Picrate*	*Acetyl deriv.*	*Benzoyl deriv.*
m-Nitroaniline			114		143	155	157
p-Nitroaniline			148		100	216	199
1-Naphthylamine			50		163	160	161
2-Naphthylamine			113		195	134	162
1-Phenylethylamine				187	190	57	120
2-Phenylethylamine				198	172	–	116
o-Phenitidine				227	158	79	104
m-Phenitidine				248	–	96	103
p-Phenitidine				254	70	138	173
o-Phenylene-diamines			102		208	186	303
m-Phenylene-diamines			64		184	191	240
p-Phenylene-diamines			141		–	304	300
o-Toluidine				200	214	112	143
m-Toluidine				203	195	66	125
p-Toluidine				200	181	152	158
2,3,6-Trichloro-aniline			78		83	206	174
2,4,6-Tribromo-aniline			120		–	238	198

Table 4.8 : Secondary amines and their derivatives

Name of the compound	Aliphatic		Aromatic		Derivatives m.p. °C		
	m.p.	b.p.	m.p.	b.p.	Picrate deriv.	Acetyl deriv.	Benzoyl deriv.
N-Benzylaniline			38	306	48	58	107
Carbazole			238		185	69	98
Diethylamine		56			155	186	–
Di-n-propylamine		111			75	210	–
Di-iso-propylamine		84			140	–	–
Di-n-butylamine		159			59	–	–
Dibenzylamine				300	–	93	112
Diphenylamine		54		302	182	103	180
Di-p-tolylamine		79		330	–	85	125
N-Ethylaniline				205	138	54	60
N-Methylaniline				194	145	103	63
Morpholine				130	148	–	75
N-n-propylaniline				222	–	47	–
Pyrrolidine		89			112	–	–
Piperidine		105		–	152	–	48
Piperizine hexahydrate	44						
Piperizine	104	145			280	144	196
Tetrahydroquinoline				250	142	–	76

Table 4.9 : Tertiary amines and their derivatives

Name of the compound	*Aliphatic*		*Aromatic*		*Derivatives m.p. °C*
	m.p.	*b.p.*	*m.p.*	*b.p.*	*Picrate*
Acridine				111	208
N,N-Dimethyl-O-toluidine				185	122
N,N-Dimethyl-m-toluidine				212	131
N,N-Dimethyl-m-toluidine				211	130
N,N-Dimethyl-1-naphthylamine				273	145
N,N-Dimethyl-2-naphthylamine			47	305	206
2,4-Dimethyl pyridine (lutidine)				129	170
2,6-Dimethyl pyridine (lutidine)				157	183
2-Methyl pyridine (2-picoline)				129	170
3-Methyl pyridine (3-picoline)				144	150
4-Methyl pyridine (4-picoline)				143	167
N,-N-Diethylaniline				215	142
N-Ethyl, n-methylaniline				201	134
N,N-Dibenzylaniline			70	300	132
Pyridine			80	115	167

(*contd.*)

Table 4.9

Name of the compound	Aliphatic		Aromatic		Derivatives m.p. °C
	m.p.	*b.p.*	*m.p.*	*b.p.*	*Picrate*
Triethylamine		90			173
Tri-n-propylamine		156			117
Tri-n-butylamine		216			106
Tribenzylamine			92		190
Tri-phenylamine			127		(Form no picrate trinitro-derivative, m.p. 280°)
Quinoline				238	203
Isoquinoline	242 223				

Table 4.10 : Hydrocarbons and their derivatives

Name of the organic compounds	*m.p. °C*		*Derivatives and their m.p. °C*		
	Aliphatic	*Aromatic*	*Nitro position of nitro group*	*Picrate*	*Bromo*
Solids					
Dibenzyl		52	4,4′ dinitro-180	100	–
Diphenyl		69	4,4′ dinitro-237	–	4,4′ dibromo 169
Naphthalene		80	1 nitro-61	149	– (Phthalic acid-195)
Phenanthrene		98	–	144	
Stilbene		125	–	95	Dibromo 237
Anthracene		216	–	138	–
Triphenyl methane		92	4,4′,4″ trinitro-206	–	Monobromo 152

(contd.)

Table 4.10

Name of the organic compound	*b.p. °C*		*Derivatives and their m.p. °C*		
	Aliphatic	*Aromatic*	*Nitro position of nitro group*	*Picrate*	*Bromo*
Liquids					
Benzene		80	1,3 dinitro 90	84	1,4 dibromo 89
Toluene		111	2,4, dinitro 70	88	– (Benzoic acid-121)
o-Xylene		144	4,5 dinitro 71	81	Monobromo 76
m-Xylene		139	2,4 dinitro 82 2,4,6 trinitro 183	91	Monobromo 76
p-Xylene		138	2,3,5 trinitro 139	90	Monobromo 144
Ethylbenzene		136	2,4,6 trinitro 37	96	
Diphenylmethane		261	2,4,2′4′ tetranitro 172		

(c) Sulphonyl Chlorides

$$ArSO_3H + PCl_5 \longrightarrow \underset{\text{(Sulphonyl chloride)}}{Ar{\cdot}SO_2Cl} + POCl_3 + HCl$$

1 g of organic compound + 2 g PCl_5, grind till it becomes liquid or semi solid. Warm it on a water bath for 5-10 minutes. Add excess water and extract the sulphonyl chloride with water. Evaporate ether and collect the residue. Determine its m.p.

*Sulphonic acids may be present as their alkali metal salts and hence, their m.p.'s are not very reliable. Moreover, these acids are hygroscopic in nature. So, these acids can be identified by converting them into sulphonamide or sulphonanilide crystalline derivatives and have sharp m.p.'s.

11. DERIVATIVES OF AMIDES, IMIDES AND ANILIDES

The best method for derivative preparation of this group is the hydrolysis of the given organic compound and then identify the hydrolytic products.

$$RCONH_2 + HCl \xrightarrow{H_2O} RCOOH + NH_4Cl$$

$$RCONHR' + NaOH \xrightarrow{H_2O} RCOONa + R'NH_2$$

Alkaline hydrolysis is faster than acid hydrolysis.

(a) Identification of Hydrolytic Products

Take 2 g of organic compound + 25 ml of 10% NaOH solution. Boil for half an hour, cool in ice + conc. HCl dropwise till strongly acidic. Acid would separate out as a solid. Filter, recrystalize from alcohol and find m.p.

(b) Picrates

Procedure is same as given for the preparation of picrates of hydrocarbons.

Table 4.11 : Sulphonic acids and their derivatives

Name of the compound	*Aliphatic*		*Aromatic*		*Derivatives and their m.p. °C*		
	m.p. (°C)	*b.p. (°C)*	*m.p. (°C)*	*b.p. (°C)*	*Sulphonamide*	*Sulphonanilide*	*Sulphonyl chloride*
Benzene sulphonic acid			65	–	153	110	–
Benzene-o-disulphonic acid			–	–	254	241	143
Benzene-m-disulphonic acid			–	–	229	144	63
Benzene-p-disulphonic acid			–	–	288	249	141
Naphthalene-1-sulphonic acid			85-90°	–	150	112	68
Naphthalene-2-sulphonic acid			124	–	217	132	79
Sulphanilic acid			decomp above 300°		164	200	–
Toluene-o-sulphonic acid			57		156	170	68
Toluene-p-sulphonic acid			92		137	103	71
Toluene-m-sulphonic acid			–		108	96	–

Table 4.12 : Amides and their derivatives

Name of the compound	*Aliphatic*		*Aromatic*		*Derivatives and their m.p. °C*	
	m.p.	*b.p.*	*m.p.*	*b.p.*	*Acids*	
Acetamide	82				–	(Picrates m.p. 107)
Benzamide	129				121	–
o-Bromobenzamide			155		150	
p-Bromobenzamide			189	252		
o-Chlorobenzamide			141		141	
p-Chlorobenzamide			179		243	
Salicylamide			139		158	
Succinamide	260				185	
o-Toluamide			143		105	
m-Toluamide			95		111	
p-Toluamide			159		178	

(*contd.*)

Table 4.12

Name of the compound	Aliphatic		Aromatic		Derivatives and their m.p. °C	
	m.p.	b.p.	m.p.	b.p.	Acids	
Urea*	132				–	(Urea nitrate 163° Urea oxalate 171°)
Thiourea**	182				–	(Benzyl thiouronium chloride m.p. 170-174°)

* *Preparation of urea nitrate.*
Dissolve 1 g of organic compound (urea) in 5 ml water + 3-4 ml conc. HNO_3 + Boil, Cool, white crystals of urea nitrate are obtained, m.p. 163°.

* *Preparation of urea oxalate.*
Dissolve 1 g of organic compound in 5 ml water + 1.2 g oxalic acid in 5 ml water. On stirring with a glass rod, the oxalate crystallizes out.

** *Derivatives of Thiourea* (Benzylthiouronium chloride)
1 g organic compound (thiourea)
+ 2 ml (or 2.2 g) Benzyl chloride + 3 ml ethanol. Warm on a water bath with shaking and then boil under reflux for 30 minutes. Cool in ice water.
Filter the solid crystals, wash it with ethyl acetate.
Yield 2 g, m.p. 170-174°C.

12. HALOGENO-HYDROCARBONS

The analysis of halogen containing organic compounds is done in the following way :

(i) To detect the presence of halogen (Cl, Br or I).
(ii) To determine m.p. or b.p. of the given organic compound.
(iii) To prepare a suitable derivative.

The ignition test is inconclusive in highly halogenated aliphatic compounds, which burn with sooty flame, e.g. chloral hydrate, $CHCl_3$, etc.

To decide the aromatic or aliphatic nature, the organic compound is hydrolysed with alcoholic NaOH.

1 ml (or 1 g) of organic compound (which contains halogen) + 10 ml alcoholic NaOH. Reflux it for 10 minutes. Take a small portion of the above mixture. Dilute it with water + dil. HNO_3 until acidic + $AgNO_3$ solution $\longrightarrow$ AgCl ppt. is produced, if compound is aliphatic or aromatic containing halogen in the side chain.

If no ppt. or very light turbidity appears, then the given organic compound is aromatic. A further confirmation is done by nitration. Only aromatic halogen compounds would undergo nitration.

NITRATION

Take 1 ml of organic compound (chlorobenzene, bromobenzene, iodobenzene, benzyl chloride) + 2 ml conc. HNO_3 + 2 ml conc. H_2SO_4. Warm very slowly with continuous shaking for 5 minutes. Pour into 30 ml water. Scratch with a glass rod, an oil solidifies to a pale yellow crystalline mass.

Name	*b.p. °C*	*Derivative*	*m.p. °C*
Chloro benzene	132	2,4-Dinitro	52
Bromo benzene	156	2,4-Dinitro	75
Iodo benzene	188	p-nitro	174
Benzyl chloride	179	p-nitro	71

OXIDATION TO BENZOIC ACID

Take 1 ml of organic compound (Benzyl chloride, o, m and p-chlorotoluene) + 30 ml saturated aq. $KMnO_4$ solution + 2 g anhydrous Na_2CO_3. Reflux for 30 minutes. Acidify with conc. HCl + 20% Na_2SO_3 solution until the brown ppt. of MnO_2 dissolves. Cool, solid crystallizes out. Filter, recrystallize from water, determine m.p.

Name	*b.p. °C*	*Derivative*	*m.p. °C*
Benzyl chloride	179	Benzoic acid	121
o-Chloro toluene	159	o-Chlorobenzoic acid	140
m-Chloro toluene	162	m-Chlorobenzoic acid	153
p-Chlorotoluene	162	p-Chlorobenzoic acid	162

Chloroform, Iodoform, CCl_4 gives isocyanide reaction (carbylamine test)

1 ml (or 0.5 g) of organic compound (chloroform, iodoform or CCl_4) + 2 ml aq. NaOH + 1 ml ethanol + 3 drops of aniline. Mix well and warm. Fowl odour of isocyanide is produced.

(Cool immediately + excess of conc. HCl to hydrolyse isocyanide to the odourless amine.)

SPECIAL TESTS

(i) Chloroform

(a) Gives isocyanide reaction.
(b) 0.2 g resorcinol + 1 ml 30% NaOH solution + 1 ml chloroform. Warm gently. Aq. layer turns red and shows a slight flourescence.
(c) The above test (b) with β-naphthol in place of resorcinol gives deep blue colour which fades to green.

(ii) Iodoform

(a) Gives isocyanide reaction
(b) On heating, iodoform gives violet vapours of iodine.

(iii) CCl_4

(a) Gives isocyanide reaction.

Table 4.13 : Halogens hydrocarbons and their derivatives

Name	*Aliphatic*		*Aromatic*		*Derivative m.p. °C*	
	m.p.	*b.p.*	*m.p.*	*b.p.*	*Acid derivatives*	*Nitro*
Benzyl chloride				179	Benzoic acid-121	p-Nitro 71
Benzy1 bromide				198	Benzoic acid-121	
Benzyl iodide			24		Benzoic acid-121	
o-Bromo toluene				181	o-Bromobenzoic acid-150	
m-Bromo toluene				183	m-Bromobenzoic acid-155	
p-Bromo toluene				185	p-Bromobenzoic acid-252	
1-Bromo naphathalene				281	–	–
2-Bromo naphathalene				281	–	–
Bromoform				151	–	–
Bromo benzene				156	–	2,4-Dinitro 75
Chloroform		61			–	–
Carbon tetrachloride		77		–	–	
Chloro benzene				132	–	2,4-Dinitro 52
o-Chlorotoluene				159	o-Chlorobenzoic acid 140	
m-chlorotoluene				162	m-Chlorobenzoic acid 158	
o-Dichloro benzene				179	–	4,5-Dinitro 110
m-Dichloro benene				172	–	4,6-Dinitro 103
p-Dichloro benzene			53			
Iodoform	120					
Iodobenzene				188	–	p-Nitro 174
p-chlorotoluene				162	p-Chlorobenzoic acid 243	

CHAPTER

5

Identification Tests for Sulphonamides, Barbiturates, Phenothiazines and Antibiotics

SULPHAZIAZINE

Aim: To identify the given sample of sulphadiazine.

Structural Formula

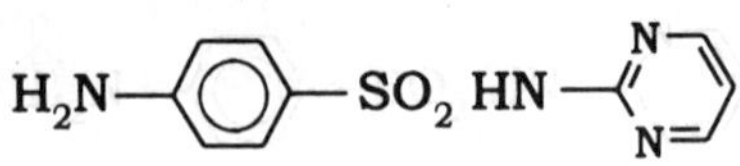

Solubility

(a) In water - insoluble.
(b) In alcohol and acetone it is separingly soluble.
(c) In dilute mineral acids - it is freely soluble.
(d) In aqueous solutions of alkali hydroxides it is freely soluble.

Colour : White, pinkish white or yellow white crystals or powder.

Odour : Odourless.

Taste : Tasteless.

Melting Range : 252-256°C (with decomposition)

Category : Antibacterial.

Identification Tests

(a) Take 5 ml water + 2 ml of 0.1 N NaOH + 50 mg of the substance (sulphadiazine). Shake until it dissolves +0.5 ml copper sulphate solution; an olive-green ppt., which becomes purple grey on standing.

(b) Take 50 mg of the substance (sulphadiazine) in a dry test tube. Heat until it melts; a reddish brown colour appears. Place moistened lead acetate paper on the mouth of the test tube during heating. Fumes do not discolour lead acetate paper (distinction from succinyl sulphathiazole).

(c)

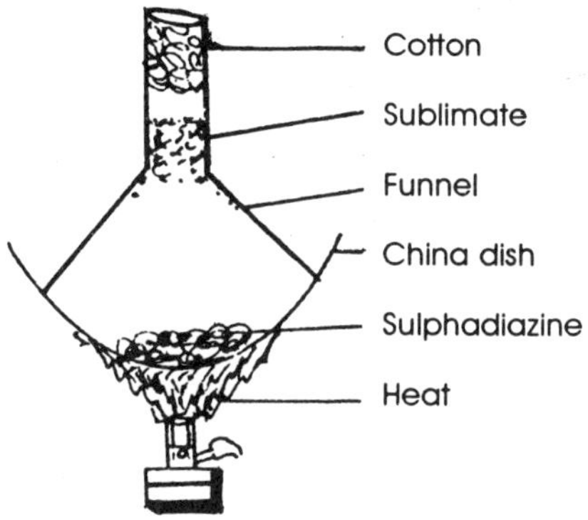

Fig. 5.1: Identification Test

Take 1 g of the substance in a china dish (porcelain dish). Place an inverted small funnel over the dish as shown in Fig. 5.1. Heat gently until a sublimate is deposited at the walls of the funnel. Collect the sublimate in a test tube. Add 1 ml of 5% resorcinol in alcohol (0.5 g resorcinol in 10 ml ethanol) + 1 ml H_2SO_4. Shake, a deep red colour appears at once + 25 ml ice cold water + 10 ml dilute ammonia solution; a blue or reddish blue colour is produced.

(d) 0.1 g of the substance + 5 ml of 1 N NaOH solution. Heat on a boiling water bath for 30 min., cool + 5 ml water. Neutralise with dil. HCl, ppts are formed. Filter, wash with water and dry the ppts.

Melting range of the residue : 198-202°C.

SULPHACETAMIDE

Aim : To identify the given sample of sulphacetamide sodium.

Structural Formula

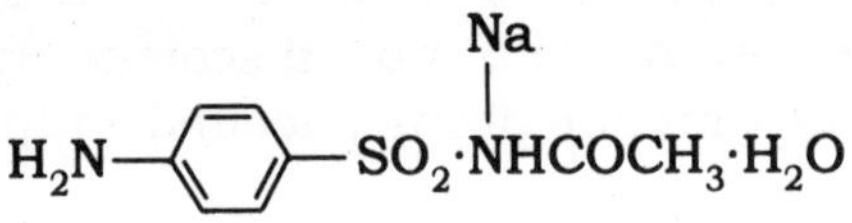

Solubility

(a) In chloroform and benzene - insoluble.
(b) In alcohol - sparingly soluble.
(c) In water - freely soluble in water.

Colour : White or yellowish white powder.

Odour : Odourless.

Taste : Bitter.

Category : Antibacterial.

Identification Tests

(a) Dissolve 1 g of the substance in 10 ml water + 2 ml acetic acid. A white or yellowish white precipitate of sulphacetamide is produced. Filter, wash it with cold water. Dry it. Determine m.p. (literature value : 182-184°C).

(b) Heat the sulphacetamide obtained in part (a) with conc. H_2SO_4 and alcohol; ethyl acetate is produced which is recognizable by its odour.

(c) In test tube no. 1, dissolve 0.1 g of sulphacetamide obtained in part (a) In 2 ml of warm dil. HCl. Cool in ice + 2 ml sodium nitrite solution. Cool again.

In test tube no. 2, dissolve 1 g sodium acetate in 2 ml of β-naphthol solution. Mix the contents of test tube no. 1 and 2; an orange ppt. is produced.

PHTHALYLSULPHATHIAZOLE

Aim : To identify the given sample of phthalylsulphathiazole.

Structural Formula

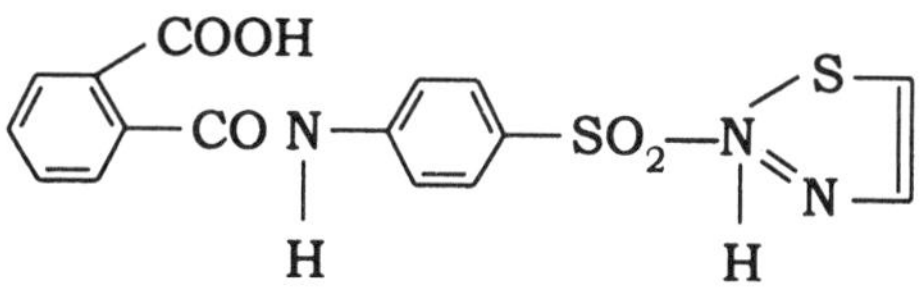

Solubility

(a) In water - insoluble.
(b) In alcohol - slightly soluble.
(c) In dil. HCl - soluble.
(d) In alkali hydroxides solutions - soluble.

Colour : White or yellowish white powder

Odour : Odourless.

Taste : Slightly bitter.

Melting Range : Darkens at 250°C and melts at 274-276°C with decomposition.

Category : Antibacterial.

Identification Tests

(a) Take 0.5 g of the substance in a dry test tube. Heat strongly. Place a lead acetate moistened paper on the mouth of the test tube during heating. Paper turns black.

(b) Dissolve 2 g of the substance in 10 ml of 5% NaOH. Boil it for 5 minutes. Cool, +15 ml dil. HCl. Add slowly 5% $NaHCO_3$ solution in water until no more CO_2 is evolved and a white ppt. forms. Filter, wash it with water. Dry it. Determine its m.p.°C (literature value 200-202°C).

(c) Take 0.1 g of the substance + 0.1 g of resorcinol + 1 ml conc. H_2SO_4. Heat for 2 minutes. Cool, pour into water and make alkaline with 10% NaOH solution; the solution obtained shows a green flourescence. The fluorescence disappears, when the solution is made acidic but reappears when it is made alkaline.

AMYLOBARBITONE

Aim : To identify the given sample of amylobarbitone.

Structural Formula

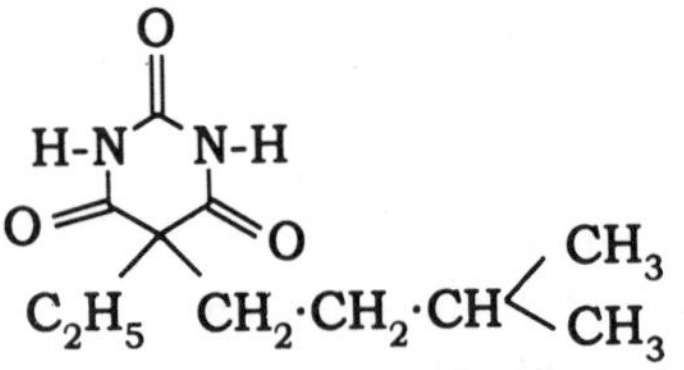

(Amylobarbitone)
or
(5-ethyl-5-isopentylbarbituric acid)

Solubility

(a) In water - slightly soluble.
(b) In alcohol - freely soluble.
(c) In chloroform - soluble.
(d) Aq. soln. of alkali hydroxides and carbonates soluble.

Colour : White.
Taste : Slightly bitter.
Odour : Odourless.
Melting range : 156-159°C.
Category : Hypnotic sedative.

Identification Tests

(a) Dissolve 0.1 g of the substance in 1 ml of 1 N NaOH + 2 ml pyridine, shake. Further add 5 ml pyridine + 1 ml copper sulphate solution in pyridine. Wait for 10 minutes. A reddish-violet ppt. is produced.

(b) Dissolve 0.1 g of the substance in 3 ml of 0.2% solution of cobalt acetate in Methanol (0.02 g of cobalt acetate in 10 ml methanol) + Powdered borax. Heat to boiling. A bluish-violet colour is produced.

(c) Take 0.5 g of the substance + 10 ml of NaOH solution. Boil it. Ammonia is evolved.

(d) Take 0.5 g of the substance + 3 ml of IN NaOH solution. + 2 ml water + 0.5 g of 4-nitrobenzyl bromide (or 4-nitrobenzyl chloride) in 10 ml of alcohol. Reflux it for half on hour. Cool, filter the ppt., wash it with water. Dry it. Determine m.p.°C.

Literature value : 150-154°C (lower melting range)
or
168-172°C (higher melting range)

AMYLOBARBITONE SODIUM

Aim : To identify the given sample of amylobarbitone sodium.

Structural Formula

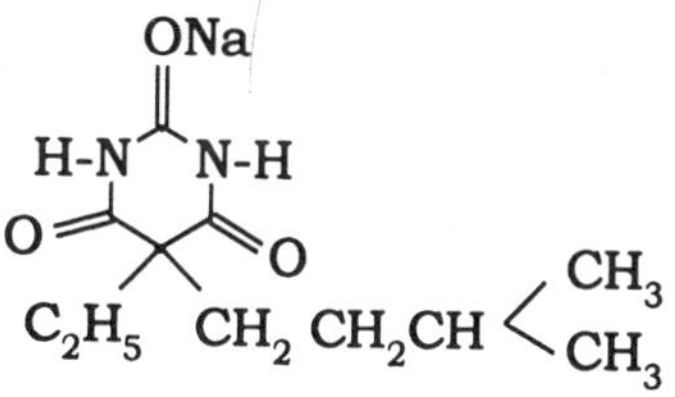

(Amylobarbitone Sodium)

Solubility

(a) In water - soluble.
(b) In alcohol - soluble.
(c) In chloroform - insoluble.
(d) In solvent ether - insoluble.

Colour : White, granular, hygroscopic powder.

Taste : Bitter.

Odour : Odourless.

Category : Hypnotic, sedative.

Identification Tests

(a) Dissolve 1 g of the substance in 15 ml water + 2 ml conc. HCl, shake and extract the amylobarbitone four times with 20 ml chloroform. Evaporate the filterate on a water bath. Dry the residue. Determine its m.p. (Literature value 156-159°C).
The residue also responds to identification tests (a) to (d) described under Amylobarbitone.

PHENOTHIAZINES

Aim : To identify a given sample of chlorpromazine hydrochloride.

Structural Formula

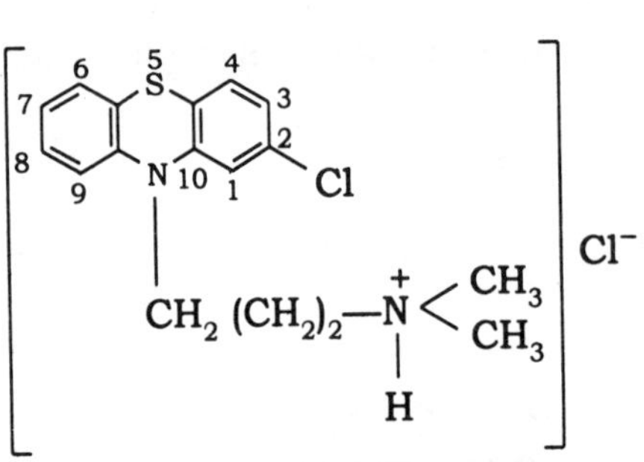

2-Chloro-10-(3-dimethyl aminopropyl
phenothiazine hydrochloride)
or
(Chlorpromazine)
hydrochloride

Solubility

(a) In water - soluble.
(b) In alcohol - soluble.

(c) In chloroform - soluble
(d) In solvent ether - insoluble

Colour : White or creamy white powder.

Odour : Odourless.

Taste : Very bitter.

Melting range : 194-198°C.

Category : Central depressant, Tranquilliser.

Identification Tests

(a) Dissolve 10 mg of the substance in 5 ml conc. H_2SO_4; a cherry red colour is produced, which darkens slowly on standing.
Take a small portion of this solution and warm it; colour changes from brown to magenta.
Take the remaining portion and add 0.5 ml of 0.1 N $K_2Cr_2O_7$; colour changes to brownish red.

(b) Dissolve 5 mg of the substance in 5 ml water +1 drop of ferric chloride solution; a stable red colour is produced.

(c) Dissolve 5 mg of the substance in 5 ml water + 0.5 ml dil. HNO_3, a red colour and a transient white turbidity is produced. The colour quickly deepens and after some time the solution becomes colourless.

AMPICILLIN

Aim : To identify the given sample of ampicillin.

Structural Formula

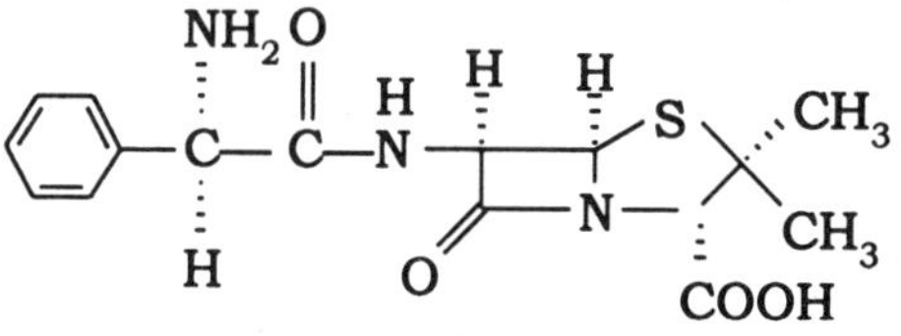

Solubility

(a) In water - slightly soluble.
(b) In alcohol - insoluble.

(c) In chloroform - insoluble.
(d) Solvent ether - insoluble.

Colour : White.

Odour : Odourless.

Taste : Bitter.

Category : Antibacterial.

Identification Tests

(a) Place 0.1 ml of a 0.1% w/v solution of ninhydrin on a filter paper; dry it. Superimpose 0.1 ml of a 0.1% of the substance being examined; Heat for 2 minutes and allow to cool; a mauve colour is obtained.
(b) Suspend 10 mg in 1 ml of water, +2 ml of potassium cupri-tartarate + 6 ml water; a magenta-violet colour is produced.

PROCAINE BENZYL PENICILLIN

Aim : To identify the given sample of procaine benzyl penicillin.

Structural Formula

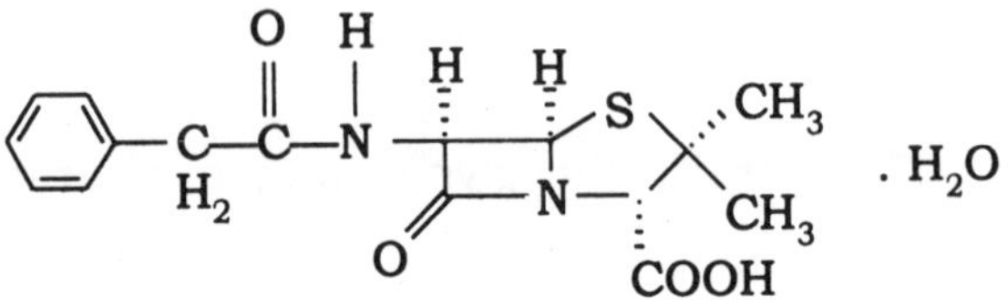

Solubility

(a) In water - slightly soluble.
(b) In alcohol - soluble.
(c) In saline solution - soluble.

Colour : White crystalline powder.

Odour : Colourless.

Taste : Almost tasteless.

Category : Antibiotic.

Identification Tests

(a) Dissolve 0.1 g of the substance in 2 ml dil. HCl, heat if necessary and cool in ice + 4 ml cooled sodium nitrite solution, and pour the mixture in 3 ml ice cooled solution of β-naphthol containing 1 g sodium acetate; a bright orange-red precipitate is produced.

CHLORAMPHENICOL

Aim: To identify the given sample of Chloramphenicol.

Structural Formula

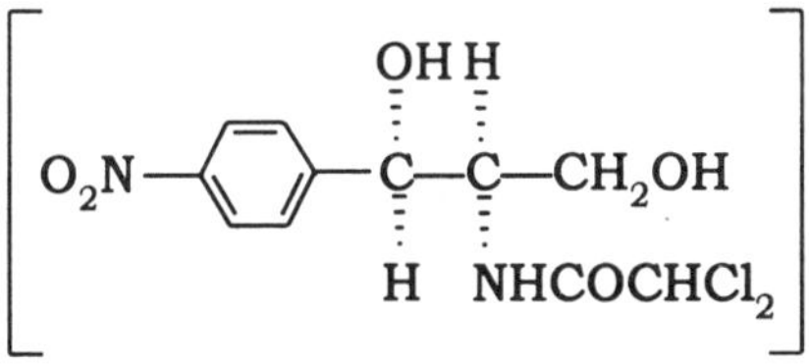

$C_{11}H_{12}Cl_2N_2O_5$ Mol. Wt. 323.13

Chloramphenicol is 2, 2-dichloro-N-[að-R,b-R)- b55D-hydroxy-að-hydroxymethyl -4-nitrophenethyl] acetamide. It is produced by the growth of certain strains of Streptomyces venezuelae in a suitable medium, but is normally prepared by synthesis.

Category: Antibacterial.

Dose: For an adult, 1.5 to 3 g daily, in divided doses; for a child, 25 to 50 mg per kg of body weight daily, in divided doses.

Description: White to greyish-white or yellowish-white, fine crystalline powder or fine-crystals, needles or elongated plates; odourless.

Solubility: Freely soluble in ethanol (95%) and in 1, 2-propanediol; slightly soluble in water and in ether.

Storage: Store in tightly-closed, light resistant containers. If the material is intended for use in the manufacture of injectable or ophthalmic preparations without further appropriate procedure of sterilisation, the container should be sterile, tamper-evident and sealed so as to exclude mirco-organisms.

Labelling: The label states whether or not the contents are intended for use in the manufacture of injectable or ophthalmic preparations.

Standards: Chloramphenicol contains not less than 98.0 per cent and not more than 102.0 per cent of $C_{11}H_{12}CI_2N_2O_5$, calculated with reference to the dried substance.

Identification Tests: Test A may be omitted if tests B, C, D and E are carried out. Tests B, C and D may omitted if tests A and E are carried out.

A: The infra-red absorption spectrum, is concordant with reference spectrum of chloramphenicol or with the spectrum obtained from chloramphenicol RS.

B: In the test for **Related substances**, the principal spot in the chromatogram obtained with solution (1) corresponds to that in the chromatogram obtained with solution (2).

C: Dissolve 10 mg in 1 ml of ethanol (50%), add 3 ml of a 1% w/v solution of calcium chloride and 50 mg of zinc powder and heat on a water-bath for 10 minutes. Decant the clear supernatant liquid into a test-tube, add 0.1 g of anhydrous sodium acetate and 0.1 ml of benzoyl chloride, shake for 1 minute and add 0.5 ml of a 10.5% w/v solution of ferric chloride hexahydrate and, if necessary, add sufficient dilute hydrochloric acid to produce a clear solution; a red-violet to purple colour is produced. Repeat the test omitting the zinc powder; no red colour is produced.

D: Heat 50 mg with 2 ml of ethanolic potassium hydroxide solution in covered test-tube on a water-bath for 15 minutes; the resulting solution gives the reactions of chlorides.

E: Melts between 149° and 153°.

pH: Between 4.5 and 7.5, determined in a suspension prepared by shaking 50 mg with 10 ml of carbon dioxide-free water.

Specific optical rotation: Between +17° and +20°, determined in a 5% w/v solution of ethanol.

Chloride: To 2.0 g add 20 ml of water and 10 ml of nitric acid and shake for 5 minutes. Filter through a filter paper previously washed by filtering 5-ml quantities of water until 5 ml of the filtrate is no longer opalescent on addition of 0.1 ml of nitric acid and 0.1 ml of a 4.25% w/v solution of silver nitrate. The resulting filtrate complies with the limit test for chlorides (125 ppm).

Related substances: Carry out the method for thin-layer chromatography, using silica gel GF254 as the coating substance and a mixture of 90 volumes of chloroform, 10 volumes of methanol and 1 volume of water as the mobile phase. Apply separately to the plate 1 mðl and 20 mðl of solution (1) 1 mðl of solution (2) and 20 mðl of solution (3). Solution (1) contains 1.0% w/v of the substance being examined in acetone. Solution (2) contains 1.0% u/v of chloramphenicol RS in acetone. For solution (3) dilute 0.5 ml of solution (2) to 100 ml with acetone. After removal of the plate, allow it to dry in air and examine under ultra-violet light (254nm). Any secondary spot in the chromatogram obtained with 2 mðl of solution (1) is not more intense than the spot in the chromatogram obtained with solution (3).

Sulphated ash: Not more than 0.1%.

Loss on drying: Not more than 0.5%, determined on 1 g by drying in an oven at 105°.

Assay: Weigh accurately about 0.125 g an dissolve in sufficient water to produce 250.0 ml. Dilute 10.0 ml with sufficient water to produce 250.0 ml. Measure the absorbance of the resulting solution at the maximum at about 278 nm. Calculate the content of $C_{11}H_{12}CI_2N_2O_5$ taking 297 as the value A (1%, 1 cm) at the maximum at about 278 nm.

Chloramphenicol intended for use in the manufacture of injectable preparations complies with the following additional requirement.

Pyrogens: Complies with the test for pyrogens, using 2 ml of a 0.25% w/v solution in water for injection per kg of the rabbit's weight.

Chloramphenicol intended for use in the manufacture of injectable or ophthalmic preparations without a further sterilisation procedure complies with the following additional requirement.

Sterility: Complies with the tests for sterility.

TETRACYCLINE HYDROCHLORIDE

Aim : To identify the given sample of tetracycline hydrochloride.

Structural Formula

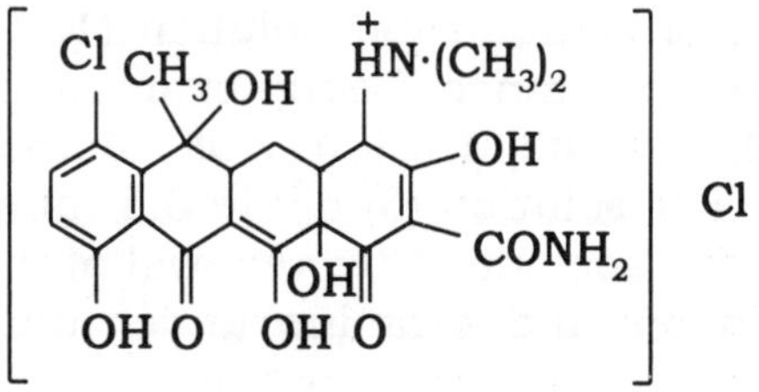

Solubility

(a) In water - soluble.
(b) In alcohol - slightly soluble.
(c) In chloroform - insoluble.
(d) In solvent ether - insoluble.

Colour : Yellow crystalline powder.

Odour : Odourless

Taste : Bitter.

Category : Antibiotic, Antiamoebic.

Identification Tests

(a) 50 mg of the substance + 3 ml conc. H_2SO_4: violet colour is produced + 2 ml water along the side of the test tube. Shake, the colour changes to deep yellow.

(b) Dissolve 50 mg of the substance in 5 ml water + $AgNO_3$ solution; white curdy precipitate is produced, soluble in dil. ammonia solution and insoluble in nitric acid.

ACETYL SALICYLIC ACID

Aim : To identify the given sample of acetyl salicylic acid (aspirin).

Structural Formula

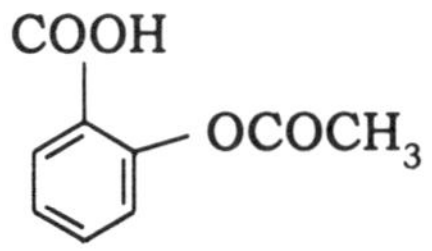

Solubility

(a) In water - slightly soluble.
(b) In alcohol - soluble.
(c) In chloroform - soluble.
(d) In solvent ether - soluble.

Colour : White or colourless crystalline powder.

Odour : Odourless.

Taste : Slightly acidic.

Melting range : 136-138°C.

Category : Analgesic.

Identification Tests

0.5 g of the substance + 10 ml NaOH solution. Boil for three minutes + 10 ml dil. H_2SO_4; white crystalline ppt. is produced and odour of acetic acid is precipitable. Filter, dissolve the ppt. in water and add ferric chloride solution. A deep violet colour is produced.

ASCORBIC ACID

Aim: To identify the given sample of Vitamin C; L-Ascorbic Acid

Structural Formula:

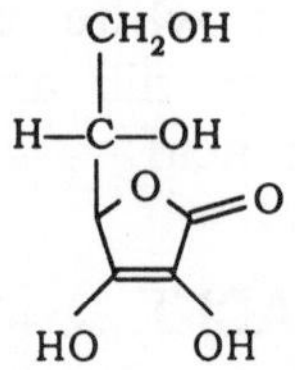

$C_6H_8O_6$ Mol. Wt. 176.13

Ascorbic Acid is (R)-5-[(S)-1, 2-dihydroxyethyl)-3, 4-dihydroxy-5 (H)-furan-2-one.

Category: Vitamin (antiscorbutic) and pharmaceutical aid (antioxidant).

Dose: Prophylactic, 25 to 75 mg daily; therapeutic, not less than 250 mg daily, in divided doses.

Description: Colourless crystals or white to very pale yellow crystalline power; odourless. On exposure to light it gradually darkens.

Solubility: Freely soluble in water; sparingly soluble in ethanol (95%); insoluble in chloroform, in ether and in benzene.

Storage: Store in tightly-closed, light-resistant containers and avoid contact with metals. It undergoes rapid decomposition in solutions in contact with air.

Standards: Ascorbic acid contains not less than 99.0 per cent and not more than 100.5 per cent of $C_6H_8O_6$.

Identification Tests

Test A may be omitted if *tests* B, C and D are carried out. *Tests* C and D may be omitted if *tests* A and B are carried out.

A: The infra-red absorption spectrum, is concordant with the reference spectrum of ascorbic acid or with the spectrum obtained from ascorbic acid RS.

B: Add 2 ml of a 2% w/v solution to a few ml of 2, 6-dichlorophenolindophenol solution; the solution is deco-lorized.

C: Dilute 1 ml of a 2% w/v solution with 5 ml of water and add 1 drop of freshly prepared 5% w/v solution of sodium nitroprusside and 2 ml of dilute sodium hydroxide solution. Add 0.6 ml of hydrochloric acid dropwise and stir; the yellow colour turns blue.

D: To 2 ml of a 2% w/v solution add 2 ml of water, 0.1 g of sodium bicarbonate and about 20 mg of ferrous sulphate, shake and allow to stand; a deep violet colour is produced. Add 5 ml of 1M sulphuric acid; the colour disappears.

pH: Between 2.2 and 2.5, determined in a 5.0% w/v solution.

Clarity and colour of solution: A 5.0% w/v solution in carbon dioxide-free water is clear, and not more intensely coloured than reference solution BYS7.

Specific optical rotation: Between +20.5° and +21.5°, determined in a 10% w/v solution, Appendix 8.9.

Light absorption: Absorbance of a 0.001% w/v solution in 0.01M hydrochloric acid at the maximum at about 244 nm, about 0.56.

Oxalic acid: Dissolve 0.25 g in 5 ml of water and neutralise to litmus paper with 2M sodium hydroxide. Add 1 ml of 2M acetic acid and 0.5 ml of 0.5M calcium chloride. Any opalescence, after 60 minutes, is not more intense than that produced by treating 5 ml of a solution prepared by dissolving 70 mg of oxalic acid in 500 ml of water in a similar manner (0.3%).

Heavy metals: Not more than 20 ppm, determined by Method A on 1.0 g dissolved in 25 ml water.

Sulphated ash: Not more than 0.1%.

Assay: Weigh accurately about 0.1 g and dissolve in a mixture of 100 ml of freshly boiled and cooled water and 25 ml of 1M sulphuric acid. Immediately titrate with 0.05M iodine, using starch solution as indicator until a persistent blue-violet colour is obtained. Each ml 0.05M iodine is equivalent to 0.008806 g of $C_6H_8O_6$.

ANALGIN

Aim: To identify the given sample of Analgin, Metamizol.

Structural Formula

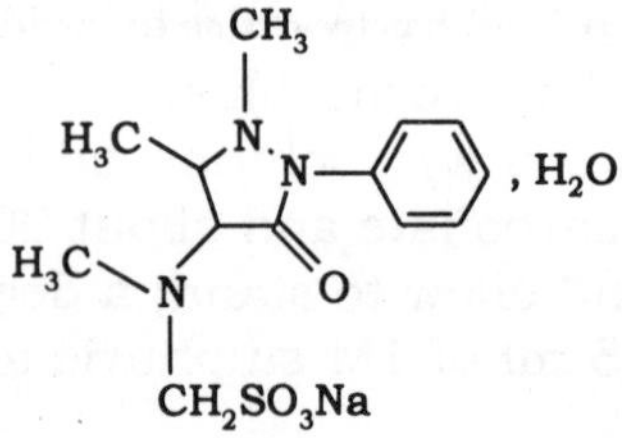

$C_{13}H_{16}N_3NaO_4S,H_2O$ Mol. Wt.351.40

Analgin is sodium [N- (2, 3-dihydro-1, 5-dimethyl-3-oxo-2-phenyl-1 H-pyrazol-4-yl)-N-methylamino] methane-sulphonate monohydrate.

Category: Analgesic.

Dose: 500 mg to 3 g daily, in divided doses.

Description: White or almost white, crystalline powder with a scarcely perceptible yellowish tinge.

Solubility: Freely soluble in water; slightly soluble in ethanol (95%); practically insoluble in chloroform and in ether.

Storage: Store in tightly-closed containers.

Standards: Analgin contains not less than 99.0 per cent not more than 100.5 per cent of $C_{13}H_{16}N_3NaO_4S$, calculated with reference to the dried substance.

Identification Tests

A: Wet about 0.1 g with two drops of water, add 5 ml of ethanol (95%) and 0.5 of dilute hydrochloric acid. To the solution add 5 ml of potassium iodate solution; a crimson colour is produced which deepens on further addition of potassium iodate solution.

B: Heat about 0.2 g with 2 ml of dilute hydrochloric acid; the characteristic odour of sulphur dioxide is produced followed by that of formaldehyde.

Acidity or alkalinity: Dissolve 0.1 g in 10 ml of freshly boiled and cooled water and add a few drops of bromothymol blue solution. Not more than 0.05 ml of 0.01M hydrochloric acid or 0.01M sodium hydroxide is required to change the colour of the solution.

Clarity of solution: A 5.0% w/v solution in water is clear.

Aminoantipyrine: Wet about 0.2 g with a few drops of water in test-tube and add 3 ml of ethanol (95%); shake until dissolved and add successively with shaking, 2 drops of dilute ammonia solution, 5 drops of potassium ferricyanide solution, 2 drops of liquefied phenol and 5 ml of water. The solution acquires a green colour gradually but not an orange or pink colour.

Heavy metals: Not more than 20 ppm, determined by Method A in a solution prepared in the following manner. Ignite 1.0 g until completely ashed. Dissolve the residue in a mixture of 23 ml of water and 2 ml of dilute acetic acid.

Arsenic: To 1.0 g in a long-necked, round-bottomed flask add 5 ml of sulphuric acid and bring to the boil gently and continue boiling on a low flame until the solution acquires a light brown colour. Cool, add dropwise about 5 ml of hydrogen peroxide solution (100 vol) and heat gently until the solution just boils and continue the heating until the solution becomes colourless. Cool and add cautiously about 20 ml of water and mix. The resulting solution complies with the limit test for arsenic, but using 0.1 ml of arsenic standard solution (10 ppm As) and dipping the stained mercuric chloride papers from the test and standard solutions in a 10% w/v solution of potassium iodide before comparison of the stains (10 ppm).

Loss on drying: Not more than 5.5%, determined on 1 g by drying in an oven at 105°.

Assay: Weigh accurately about 0.4 g, dissolve in a mixture of 40 ml of ethanol (95%) and 10 ml of 0.01M hydrochloric acid and titrate with 0.05M iodine until a yellow colour stable for 30 seconds is produced. Each ml of 0.05M iodine is equivalent to 0.01667 g of $C_{13}H_{16}N_3NaO_4S$.

ANALGIN TABLETS

Aim: To identify the given sample of Analgin—Metamizol Tablets.

Usual strength: 500 mg.

Storage: Store in tightly-closed containers.

Standards: Analgin Tablets contain not less than 95.0 per cent and not more than 105.0 per cent of the stated amount of analgin, $C_{13}H_{16}N_3NaO_4S, H_2O$.

Identification Tests: Power a few tablets and shake a quantity of the powder equivalent to about 0.5 g of Analgin with 10 ml of water and filter. The filtrate complies with the tests described under Analgin.

Other requirements: Comply with the requirements of tests stated under Tablets.

Assay: Weigh and powder 20 tablets. Weigh accurately a quantity of the powder equivalent to about 0.5 g of Analgin and transfer to a 50-ml volumetric flask. Add 10 ml of water and shake for 1 minute. Dilute to volume ethanol (95%), shake well and filter. Titrate 25.0 ml of the filtrate with 0.05M iodine until a yellow colour stable for 30 seconds is produced. Each ml of 0.05M iodine is equivalent to 0.01757 g of $C_{13}H_{16}N_3NaO_4S, H_2O$.

BENZOIC ACID

Aim: To identify the given sample of Benzoic acid.

Structural Formula

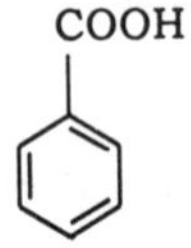

$C_7H_6O_2$ Mol. Wt. 122.12

Category: Antifungal agent; pharmaceutical aid (antimicrobial preservative).

Description: Colourless, light crystals, scales or needles; odour, slight and characteristic.

Solubility: Freely soluble in ethanol (95%), in chloroform and in ether; slightly soluble in water but soluble in boiling water. It is soluble in fixed oils.

Storage: Store in well-closed containers.

Standards: Benzoic Acid contains not less than 99.5

per cent and not more than 100.5 per cent of $C_7H_6O_2$, calculated with reference to the anhydrous substance.

Identification Tests

A: Warm gently 0.2 g with 20 ml of water, add 1 ml of 1M sodium hydroxide and filter. To the filtrate add ferric chloride test solution; a buff coloured precipitate is produced.

B: The light absorption in the range 220 to 360 mm of a 0.001% w/v solution in methanol exhibits a maximum only at about 225 nm; absorbance at about 225 nm, about 0.8.

C: A 1% w/v solution is acid to methyl red solution.

D: Melts between 121° and 123°.

Clarity and colour of solution: A 5% w/v solution in ethanol (95%) is clear and colourless..

Arsenic: Mix 5 g with 3 g of anhydrous sodium carbonate, add 10 ml of bromine solution and mix thoroughly. Evaporate to dryness on a water-bath, gently ignite and dissolve the cooled residue in 16 ml of brominated hydrochloric acid and 45 ml of water. Remove the excess of bromine with 2 ml of stannous chloride AsT. The resulting solution complies with the limit test for arsenic (2 ppm).

Heavy metals: Not more than 10 ppm, determined by the following method. Dissolve 2.0 g in 25 ml of acetone and add 2 ml of water and 10 ml of hydrogen sulphide solution; any colour produced is not more intense than that of a solution prepared with 25 ml of acetone, 2.0 ml of standard solution (10 ppm Pb) and 10 ml of hydrogen sulphide solution.

Readily oxidisable substances: Add 1 ml of sulphuric acid to 100 ml of water, heat to boiling and add dropwise 0.1M potassium permanganate until the pink colour persists for 30 seconds. Dissolve exactly 1 g in the hot solution and titrate with 0.1M potassium permanganate to a pink colour that persists for 15 seconds; not more than 0.5 ml of 0.1M potassium permanganate is required.

Readily carbonisable substances: Dissolve 0.50 g in 5 ml of sulphuric acid and allow to stand for 5 minutes. The colour of the solution is not more intense than that of reference solution YS5.

Cinnamic acid: Warm 0.1 g with 0.1 g of potassium permanganate and 5 ml of dilute sulphuric acid; no odour of benzaldehyde is developed.

Chlorinated compounds: Dissolve 0.33 g in 5 ml of 0.5M sodium carbonate, evaporate to dryness and heat the residue until completely charred, keeping the temperature below 400°. Extract the residue with a mixture of 10 ml of water and 12 ml of dilute nitric acid and filter; the filtrate complies with the limit test for chlorides.

Sulphated ash: Not more than 0.1%.

Water: Not more than 0.7% w/w, determined on 0.25 g and using a mixture of 1 volume of methanol and 2 volumes of pyridine as the solvent.

Assay: Weigh accurately about 1.0 g and dissolve in 15 ml of warm ethanol (95%) previously neutralised to phenolphthalein solution. Add 20 ml of water and titrate with 0.5M sodium hydroxide using phenolphthalein solution as indicator. Each ml of 0.5M sodium hydroxide is equivalent to 0.06106 g of $C_7H_6O_2$.

CAFFEINE

Aim: To identify the given sample of Caffeine.

Structural Formula

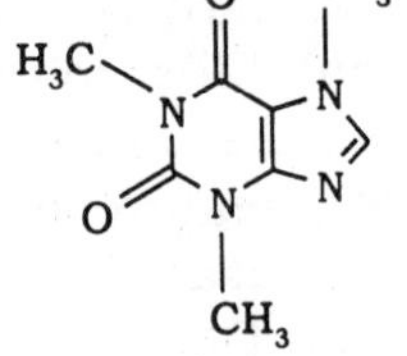

$C_8H_{10}N_4O_2$ Mol. Wt. 194.19 (anhydrous)

$C_8H_{10}N_4O_2H_20$ Mol. Wt. 212.21 (monohydrate)

Caffeine is 3, 7-dihydro-1, 3, 7-trimethyl-1H-purine 2, 6-dione or its monohydrate.

Category: Central nervous system stimulant.

Dose: 300 to 600 mg

Description: Silky white crystals or white glistening needles or white crystalline powder, odourless; sublimes readily.

Solubility: Freely soluble in chloroform and in boiling water; sparingly soluble in water and in ethanol (95%); slightly soluble in ether.

Storage: Store in tightly-closed containers.

Labelling: The label states whether it is anhydrous or monohydrate.

Standards: Caffeine contains not less than 98.5 per cent and not more than 101.5 per cent of $C_8H_{10}N_4O_2$, calculated with reference to the dried substance.

Identification Tests: Test A may be omitted if tests B, C, D and E are carried out. Tests B, C and D may be omitted if tests A and E are carried out.

A: The infra-red absorption spectrum, of the substance being examined after drying at 100° for 1 hour is concordant with the reference spectrum of caffeine or with the spectrum obtained from caffeine RS.

B: To 10 mg in a porcelain dish, add 1 ml of hydrochloric acid and 0.1 g of potassium chlorate and evaporate to dryness on a water-bath. Expose the residue to the vapours of dilute ammonia solution; a purple colour is produced which disappears on addition of a solution of a fixed alkali.

C: To a saturated solution add a few drops of tannic acid solution; a white precipitate is produced which is soluble in excess of the reagent.

D: To 5 ml of saturated solution add 1.5 ml of 0.05M iodine, the solution remains clear. Add a few drops of dilute hydrochloric acid; a brown precipitate is formed which dissolves on neutralisation with sodium hydroxide solution.

E: Melts between 234° and 239°, determined after drying at 100° for 1 hour,

Acidity or alkalinity: Dissolve 0.2 g in 10 ml of

boiling water and cool. Add 0.1 ml of bromothymol blue solution. The solution is coloured green or yellow. Titrate with 0.02M sodium hydroxide to a blue colour; not more than 0.1 ml is required.

Clarity and colour of solution: A 1.0% w/v solution is clear and colourless,

Arsenic: Mix 3.3 g with 3 g of anhydrous sodium carbonate, add 10 ml of bromine solution and mix thoroughly. Evaporate to dryness on a water-bath, gently ignite and dissolve the cooled residue in 16 ml of brominated hydrochloric acid and 45 ml of water. Remove the excess of bromine with 2 ml of stannous chloride solution AsT. The resulting solution complies with the limit test for arsenic, (3 ppm).

Heavy metals: Not more than 20 ppm, determined by Method A, on 25 ml of a solution prepared in the following manner. Mix 2.0 g with 5 ml of 0.1 M hydrochloric acid and 45 ml of water, warm gently until solution is complete and cool to room temperature.

Related substances: Carry out the method for *thin-layer chromatography,* using silica gel GF254 as the coating substance and a mixture of 40 volumes of 1-butanol, 30 volumes of chloroform, 10 volumes of strong ammonia solution and 3 volumes of acetone as the mobile phase. Apply separately to the plate 10 mðl of each of the following solutions of the substance being examined in a mixture of 3 volumes of chloroform and 2 volumes of methanol containing (1) 2.0% w/v and (2) 0.010% w/v. After removal of the plate, allow it to dry in air and examine under ultra-violet light (254 nm). Any secondary spot in the chromatogram obtained with solution (1) is not more intense than the spot in the chromatogram obtained with solution (2).

Sulphated ash: Not more than 0.1%.

Loss on drying: Not more than 0.5% (for the anhydrous form) and 8.5% (for the monohydrate form), determined on 1 g by drying at 100° for 1 hour.

Assay: Weigh accurately about 0.18 g and dissolve

with warming in 5 ml of anhydrous glacial acetic acid. For Caffeine Hydrate, use material previously dried at 100° to 105°. Cool, add 10 ml of acetic anhydride and 20 ml of toluene and carry out Method A for non-aqueous titration, determining the end-point potentiometrically. Perform a blank determination and make any necessary correction. Each ml 0.1M perchloric acid is equivalent to 0.01942 g of $C_8H_{10}N_4O_2$.

CHAPTER

6

Organic Preparations

ACETYLATION

Acetylation is the introduction of acetyl group (CH_3CO—) in place of the active hydrogen of compounds containing —OH (alcohols and phenols), —NH_2 (primary amines) and >NH (secondary amines) groups.

The acetylating reagents used for acetylation are acetyl chloride and acetic anhydride.

CH_3COCl	$(CH_3CO)_2O$
(Acetyl chloride)	(Acetic anhydride)

Acetyl chloride is used in presence of pyridine, which absorbs the HCl formed during the reaction. Acetic anhydride is used either with glacial acetic acid or fused sodium acetate.

The acetylation is very useful in:

(i) The protection of —OH or —NH_2 groups

(ii) The preparation of mono substituted derivatives of the aromatic amines or phenols.

In the protection of —OH or —NH_2 group, the first step is to convert these groups into its acetyl derivative and then perform the desirable reaction. The free —OH or —NH_2 group can be regenerated by the hydrolysis of these derivatives at the end of the reaction.

The preparation of monosubstituted derivatives of the aromatic amines or phenols cannot be prepared directly by the action of appropriate reagent, because of highly activating influence of these groups, e.g. bromination of aniline or phenol gives tribromoaniline or tribromophenol respectively, but if the amino group of aniline is protected by acetylation, the resulting compound, i.e. acetanilide, readily gives monosubstitution product, i.e. p-bromoacetanilide, which on hydrolysis gives p-bromoaniline. Similarly p-bromophenol may be prepared by protecting —OH group by acetylation, then bromination and finally by the hydrolysis gives p-bromophenol.

Experiment 1

Aim: To prepare acetanilide from aniline.

Theory: Acetyl derivatives are obtained when primary amines are treated with acetic anhydride or acetyl chloride. The mechanism of the reaction may be written as follows:

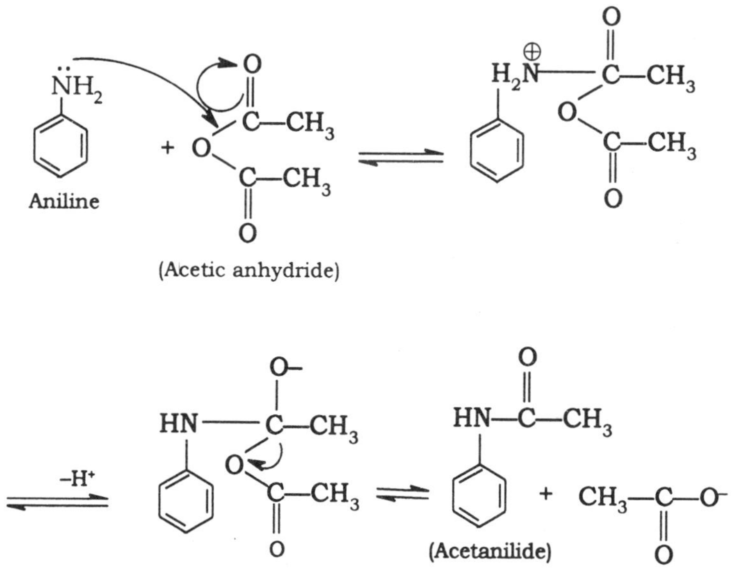

Chemicals Required

Aniline = 5 ml
Acetic anhydride = 5 ml
Glacial acetic acid = 5 ml
Ice cold water = 150 ml

Procedure

Method 1

In a 250 ml beaker, take 150 ml ice cold water. Add 5 ml of aniline with constant stirring by glass rod. Add 5 ml of acetic anhydride to it dropwise with constant stirring.

Colourless crystals of acetanilide separate out. Filter it, wash with cold water and dry by pressing it between filter papers. Recrystallise it from hot water containing 2% rectified spirit. On cooling, snow white crystals of acetanilide are obtained.

Yield = 5 g
m.p. = 114°C
Appearance = white shining flakes

Method 2

Take 5 ml aniline in a 150 ml conical flask. Add 10 ml mixture of equal volume of acetic anhydride and glacial acetic acid with shaking. Now attach the flask to a regular condenser and heat the reaction mixture for about 10 minutes under slow heating.

Cool the flask in tap water and pour the contents in a 250 ml beaker containing 150 ml cold water. Stir the solution well and filter. Wash the ppt. with cold water and recrystallise from hot water containing a little alcohol (10 ml water + 4 drops of alcohol) or from a mixture of equal volume of water and acetic acid. Filter and dry at 50-60°C. Acetanilide is obtained as colourless crystals.

Yield = 5 g
m.p. = 114°C
appearance = white shining flakes

Experiment 2

Aim: To prepare acetyl salicylic acid (Aspirin) from salicylic acid.

Theory: The phenolic group in salicylic acid can easily be acetylated with the help of acetic anhydride, in presence of concentrated sulphuric acid, to yield acetyl salicylic acid (aspirin).

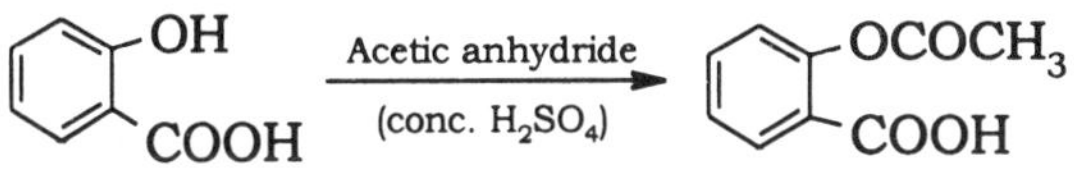

Salicylic acid (Aspirin)

Chemicals Required

Salicylic acid = 5 g
Acetic anhydride = 7 ml
Conc. sulphuric acid = 5-6 drops

Procedure

Method 1

In a 250 ml conical flask take 5 g salicylic acid, 7 ml acetic anhydride and 5-6 drops of conc. H_2SO_4. Shake the mixture throughly. Warm the reaction mixture with constant stirring on a water bath maintained at 50-60°C for about 15 minutes. Cool and then pour it in 100 ml cold water taken in a 250 ml beaker with stirring. Filter the precipitated crude product. Recrystallise from 50% acetic acid (a mixture of equal volume of water and acetic acid).

Yield = 6 g
m.p. = 136°C
Appearance = Colourless needles

Method 2

Chemicals Required

Salicylic acid = 5 g
Acetyl chloride = 4 ml
Pyridine = 4 ml

Dissolve 5 g salicylic acid in 4 ml pyridine in a 250 ml conical flask. Place the flask in ice bath. Add 4 ml of acetyl chloride dropwise with vigorous shaking. After the completion of addition of acetyl chloride, heat the reaction mixture on a boiling water bath for 10 minutes. On cooling a semi-solid mass is produced to which 100 ml ice cold water are added with stirring. Filter the solid product, wash it with cold water and dry by pressing between filter papers. Recrystallise it from a mixture of equal volumes of water and acetic acid.

Yield = 5 g
m.p. = 136°C
Appearance = Colourless needles

Method 3

Chemicals Required

Salicylic acid = 5 g
Acetic anhydride = 8 ml
Glacial acetic acid = 8 ml

Dissolve 5 g of salicylic acid in a mixture of 8 ml acetic anhydride and 8 ml glacial acetic acid taken in a 100 ml round bottom flask. Reflux the reaction mixture for about half an hour. Pour the reaction mixture in 100 ml cold water taken in a 400 ml beaker with vigorous stirring. Crystals of acetyl salicylic acid separates out. Filter it and dry by pressing between filter papers. Recrystallise it from a mixture of equal volume of water and acetic acid.

Yield = 6 g
m.p. = 136°C
Appearance = Colourless needles

BENZOYLATION

The introduction of a benzoyl group (C_6H_5CO—) in place of active hydrogen of —OH, —NH_2 or >NH group is known as benzoylation. The reagent used for benzoylation reaction is benzoyl chloride in presence of NaOH.

Benzoylation in presence of NaOH is known as Schotten-Baumann reaction.

(i) $C_6H_5OH + NaOH \longrightarrow C_6H_5ONa + H_2O$

$C_6H_5O\,\boxed{Na + Cl}\,OCC_6H_5 \longrightarrow C_6H_5O{\cdot}OC{\cdot}C_6H_5 + NaCl$

(Sodium phenoxide) (Benzoyl chloride) (Phenyl benzoate)

(ii) $C_6H_5NH_2 + C_6H_5COCl \xrightarrow{NaOH} C_6H_5NHCOC_6H_5 + HCl$

(Aniline) (Benzoyl chloride) (Benzanilide)

(iii) $R_2N\,\boxed{H + Cl}\,COC_6H_5 \xrightarrow{NaOH} R_2N\ CO\ C_6H_5 + HCl$

(N-Benzoyl derivative)

Advantages of Benzoylation Over Acetylation

(i) Benzoyl derivatives are crystalline solids with higher melting points than acetyl derivatives and have lower solubilities in most of the solvents.

(ii) Benzoyl derivatives can be easily prepared in aqueous solvents as unlike acetyl chloride or acetic anhydride, benzoyl chloride is very slowly hydrolysed by water.

Experiment

Aim: To prepare benzanilide (N-Benzoylaniline) from aniline (Schotten-Baumann reaction).

Theory: Amino compounds reacts with benzoyl chloride and gives benzoyl derivative, the reaction is known as Schotten-Baumann reaction. The mechanism of the reaction is as follows:

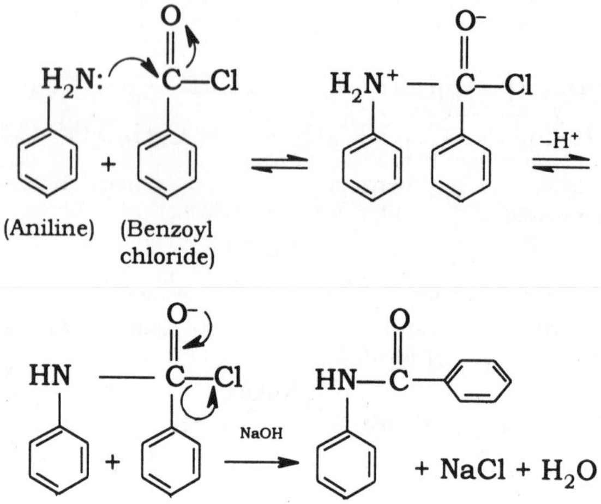

(Benzanilide)

Chemicals Required

Aniline = 5 ml

Benzoyl chloride = 7 ml

Sodium hydroxide = 10% solution (50 ml)

(Dissolve 5 g of NaOH pallets in 50 ml water)

Procedure

In a 250 ml conical flask take 5 ml aniline + 50 ml of 10% NaOH solution + 7 ml benzoyl chloride. Cork the flask and shake vigorously for 15 minutes when crude benzanilide separates out as white solid. The flask get warmed as the reaction is exothermic. The completion of the reaction is indicated by the disappearance of pungent smell of benzoyl chloride. Add about 100 ml cold water and filter the precipitated product. Wash it with cold water and recystallise from alcohol.

Yield = 9 g

m.p. = 163°C

Appearance = White crystalline solid

Experiment

Aim: To prepare phenyl benzoate from phenol.

Theory: Preparation of phenyl benzoate from phenol involves the benzoylation of phenol. This reaction is an example of Schotten-Baumann reaction.

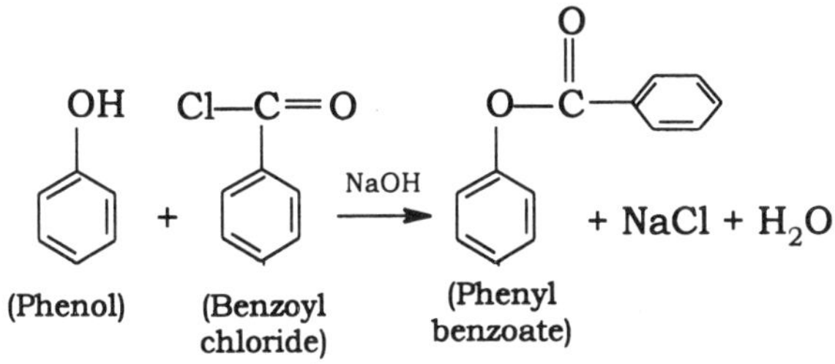

Chemicals Required

Phenol = 3 g
Benzoyl chloride = 6 ml
10% NaOH solution = 50 ml

Procedure

In a 250 ml conical flask dissolve 3 g phenol in 50 ml of 10% NaOH solution. Shake and add 6 ml benzoyl chloride. Cork the flask and shake it vigorously for about half an hour. The completion of the reaction is indicated by the disappearance of the smell of benzoyl chloride. Add 100 ml cold water to the flask. Filter the solid products obtained and wash with cold water crystallise from ethyl alcohol.

Yield = 5 g
m.p. = 69°C
Appearance = Colourless crystals

Experiment

Aim: To prepare hippuric acid (Benzoyl glycine) from glycine.

Theory: Preparation of hippuric acid from glycine involves the benzoylation of glycine at —NH_2 position.

$$H_2NCH_2COOH + C_6H_5COCl \longrightarrow C_6H_5CO{\cdot}NH{\cdot}CH_2{\cdot}COOH + HC$$

(Glycine) (Benzoyl chloride) (Hippuric acid)

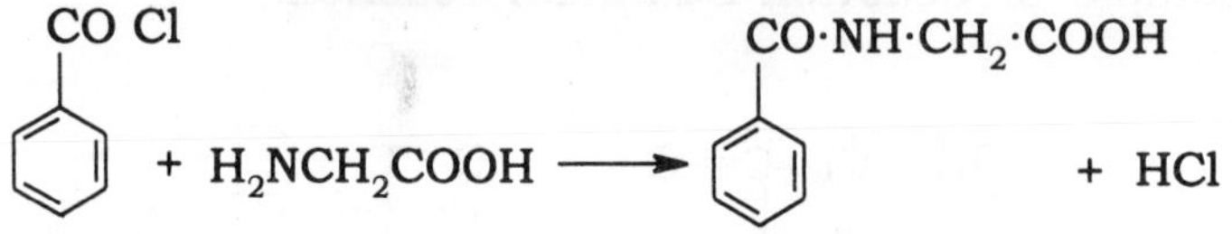

(Benzoyl chloride) (Glycine) (Hippuric acid)

Chemicals Required

(i) Glycine 5 g.
(ii) Benzoyl chloride 9 ml.
(iii) 10% NaOH solution 50 ml.
(iv) Conc. HCl.

Procedure

In a 250 ml conical flask, dissolve 5 g glycine in 50 ml of 10% NaOH solution. Add 9 ml benzoyl chloride slowly and with vigorous stirring. Cool it and add few lumps of crushed ice. Neutralise it by adding conc. HCl until the solution is just acidic to congo red paper (which turns blue on acidification). Filter the ppt. of hippuric acid. Transfer the ppt. into 250 ml beaker and add 20 ml CCl_4. Boil it for 10 minutes on a water bath. Cool it.

Hippuric acid separates out, leaving any benzoic acid formed during the reaction in solution.

Yield = 9 g
m.p. = 187°C
Appearance = White crystals

OXIDATION AND REDUCTION REACTIONS

Oxidation and reduction reactions are very common in Organic Chemistry. The definition of oxidation and reduction as Applied in Organic Chemistry is very simple.

A reaction which proceeds by the addition of oxygen is called oxidation. A reaction which proceeds by the addition of hydrogen is called reduction.

The result of oxidation and reduction depends upon the nature of the original compound and that of the reagent employed to effect the change. While reduction seldom causes a rupture of the carbon chain, oxidation does it very often.

Experiment

Aim: To prepare benzoic acid from benzyl chloride (Oxidation reaction).

Theory: Benzyl chloride on oxidation with dilute nitric acid (1 : 1 by volume) or with a mixture of potassium permanganate and sodium carbonate in aqueous solution gives benzoic acid.

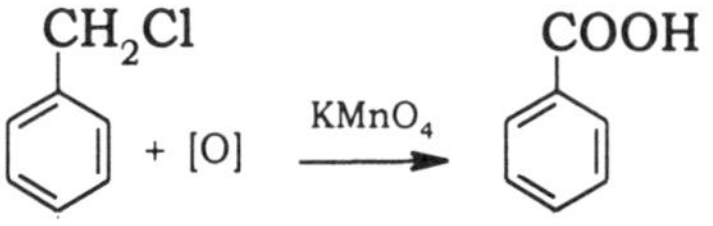

Chemicals Required

Anhydrous sodium carbonate	= 5 g
Potassium permanganate	= 10 g
Benzyl chloride	= 5 ml (5.5 g)
Sodium sulphite	= 20 g
Conc. HCl	= 50 ml

Procedure

In a 250 ml round bottom flask take 150 ml water and add in turn 5 g anhydrous sodium carbonate, 10 g of potassium permanganate and finally 5 ml of benzyl chloride. Fit the flask with a reflux water condenser. Boil the mixture gently for one hour. Now cool the flask, and add concentrated hydrochloric acid (50 ml) cautiously until the mixture is strongly acidic. Add 20% aqueous solution of sodium sulphite (100 ml) slowly with shaking until the dark brown ppt. of MnO_2 is completely dissolved and only the white ppt. of benzoic acid remains. Filter it and wash it with water. Recrystallise from boiling water.

Yield = 4.5 g
m.p. = 121°C
Appearance = Colourless needles

Experiment

Aim: To prepare benzil from benzoin.

Theory: Benzoin is oxidised by conc. HNO_3 to form benzil.

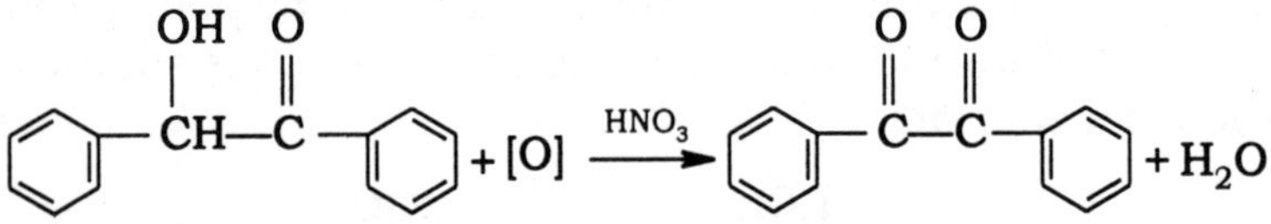

(Benzoin) (Benzil)

Chemicals Required

Benzoin = 7.5 g
Conc. HNO_3 = 40 ml
Ice

Procedure

In a 250 ml round bottom flask mix 7.5 g benzoin and 40 ml conc. HNO_3. Heat the contents on boiling water bath till the crystalline benzoin is completely replaced by an oily compound (about 2 hours). Pour the solution in 100 ml ice cold water with vigorous stirring. Filter the yellow solid and wash with water. Recrystallise from alcohol.

Yield = 7 g
m.p. = 95°C
Appearance = Pale yellow crystals

Experiment

Aim: To prepare dibenzyl from benzil (Clemmensen reduction).

Theory: The oxygen atom of the carbonyl group in an aldehyde or ketone can be replaced by hydrogen atoms through the use of amalgamated zinc and hydrochloric acid. This reaction is known as Clemmensen reduction and is used in the conversion of carbonyl groups methylene groups.

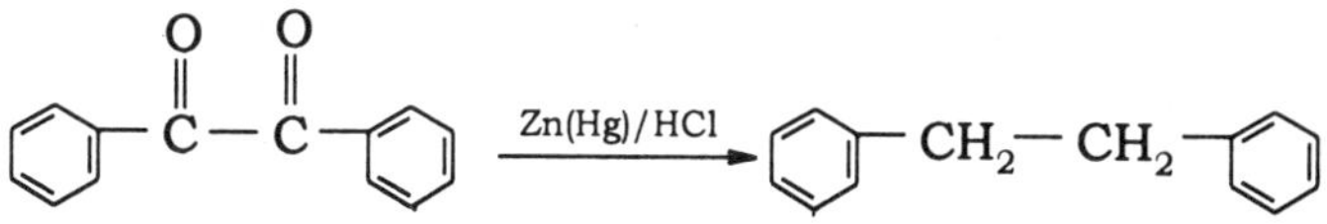

(Benzil) (Dibenzyl)

Chemicals Required

Benzil = 5 g
Zn/Hg = 20 g
Dilute HCl (50%) = 75 ml
Conc. HCl = 20 ml

Preparation of Zn/Hg amalgam

Granulated zinc or zinc foil cut in small stripes is allowed to stand for an hour in contact with an equal weight of 5% aqueous mercuric chloride solution. The contents should be frequently shaken. The solution is then pour off and the metal washed once with distilled water.

Procedure

In a 250 ml round bottom flask mix 5 g benzil, 20 g zinc amalgam and 75 ml of 50% HCl. Heat the contents under reflux water condenser for 3-4 hours. At the end of each hour add 3 ml of conc. HCl. When heating is complete, cool the liquid obtained in a ice cold water, filter the product obtained and wash with water. Recrystallise from alcohol.

Yield = 3 g
m.p. = 52°C
Appearance = Colourless crystals

Precaution: If on cooling, the product is not obtained, the liquid should first be concentrated and then cooled.

Experiment

Aim: To prepare anthraquinone from anthracene (Oxidation).

Theory: Anthracene can be oxidized to 9, 10-anthraquinone by a mixture of sodium dichromate and concentrated H_2SO_4.

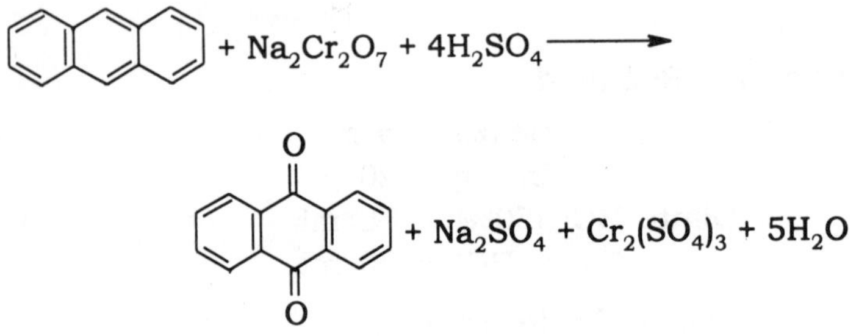

Chemicals Required

Anthracene = 5 g
Glacial acetic acid = 100 ml
$Na_2Cr_2O_7 \cdot 2H_2O$ = 13 g
Concentrated H_2SO_4 = 5 ml

Procedure

In a 250 ml round bottom flask mix 5 g anthracene and 50 ml glacial acetic acid. Boil the mixture and add slowly 13 g of sodium dichromate ($Na_2Cr_2O_7 \cdot 2H_2O$) and 5 ml concentrated H_2SO_4. Keep the temperature of reaction mixture at the boiling point. Again add 35 ml glacial acetic acid slowly in the reaction mixture over a period of 15 minutes. After the addition is complete, boil the reaction mixture for an additional 20 minutes. Cool the flask to allow the separation of solid anthraquinone. Filter it and wash it with 20 ml of 50% acetic acid and then with cold water.

Yield = 5 g
m.p. = 286°C
Appearance = Light pale yellow

Experiment

Aim: To prepare benzhydrol from benzophenone (Reduction).

Theory: Reduction of benzophenone with zinc dust and alcoholic NaOH, a mild reducing agent gives benzhydrol (a secondary alcohol).

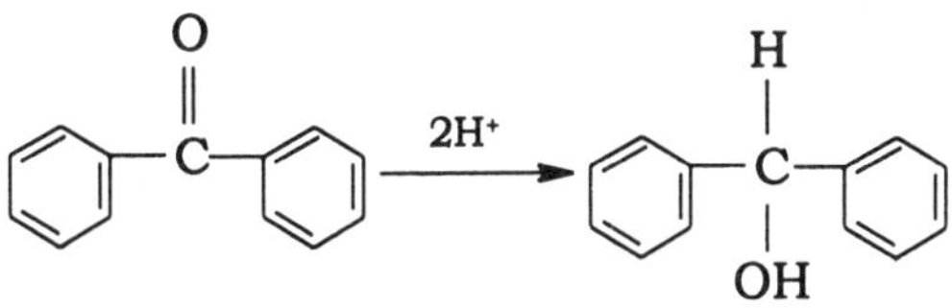

(Benzophenone) (Benzhydrol)

Chemicals Required

Benzophenone = 6 g
Ethanol = 65 ml
NaOH pallets = 6 g
Zinc powder = 6 g

Procedure

In a 250 ml round bottom flask mix 6 g benzophenone, 65 ml ethanol, 6 g NaOH pallets and 6 g zinc powder. Shake the contents and fix a reflux condenser. Warm gently on a water bath for 1 hour. Allow the flask to cool to about 60°C and then filter it. Wash the residue with 5 ml portions of ethanol two times. pour the clean filtrate in 250 ml cold water and acidify with 25 ml of concentrated HCl. A viscous oil separates out, which solidies on cooling. Recrystallise it from alcohol.

Yield = 4 g
m.p. = 68°C

OXIMES

Hydroxylamine condenses readily with aldehydes and ketones to give crystalline oximes.

$$CH_3CH\,O + H_2\,N\,OH \longrightarrow CH_3CH{=}NOH + H_2O$$

(Acetaldehyde) (Acetaldoxime)

$$\begin{matrix} CH_3 \\ CH_3 \end{matrix}\!\!>C{=}O + H_2NOH \qquad \begin{matrix} CH_3 \\ CH_3 \end{matrix}\!\!>C{=}NOH + H_2O$$

(Acetone) (Acetoxime)

Oxime formation have the following important uses:

(i) They have sharp melting points so they are used to characterize the parent aldehydes and ketones.

(ii) Impure aldehydes and ketones can be purifed by conversion into oximes, and then recrystallisation and hydrolysis of oxime gives pure aldehydes and ketones.

(iii) Reduction of oxime gives pure primary amines.

Experiment

Aim: To prepare benzophenone-oxime from benzophenone.

Theory: Hydroxylamine condenses readily with carbonyl compounds. In this preparation benzophenone oxime is obtained by condensing benzophenone with hydroxylamine.

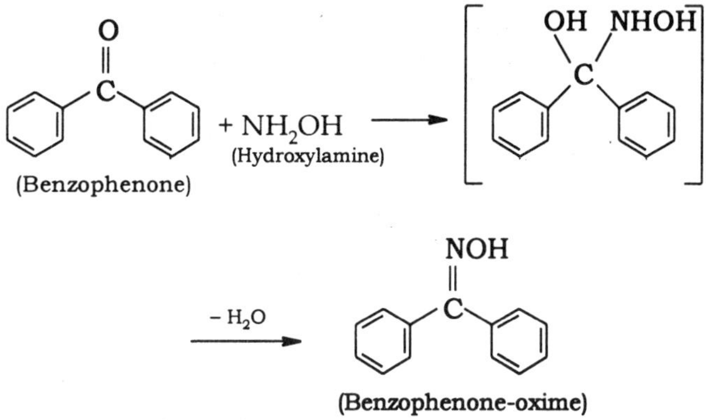

Chemicals Required

Benzophenone = 5 g
$NH_2OH \cdot HCl$ = 3 g
NaOH pallets = 6 g
C_2H_5OH = 15 ml
Conc. HCl = 15 ml

Procedure

In a 250 ml round bottom flask fitted with reflux water condenser mix 5 g benzophenone, 3 g hydroxylamine hydrochloride ($NH_2OH \cdot HCl$) and 15 ml ethanol. Shake the reaction mixture and add 6 g solid NaOH pallets in small portions at a time and then boil the reaction mixture for 10 minutes. Cool and pour the contents into 250 ml beaker containing 15 ml concentrated hydrochloric acid (conc. HCl) and 100 ml water. Filter it and wash with cold water. Recrystallise from alcohol.

Yield = 5 g
m.p. = 142°C
Appearance = Crystalline solid

ESTERIFICATION

When a monocarboxylic acid is heated with an alcohol in the presence of a small amount of mineral acid (H_2SO_4), it yields an ester and water, e.g.

$$\underset{\text{(Acetic acid)}}{CH_3COOH} + \underset{\text{(Ethanol)}}{HOC_2H_5} \rightleftharpoons \underset{\text{(Ethyl acetate)}}{CH_3COOC_2H_5} + H_2O$$

This reaction is known as esterification. If, however, conc. H_2SO_4 is present, the water is absorbed, the back reaction is prevented, and a high yield of ethyl acetate is obtained. The mechanism of the esterification involves the following steps.

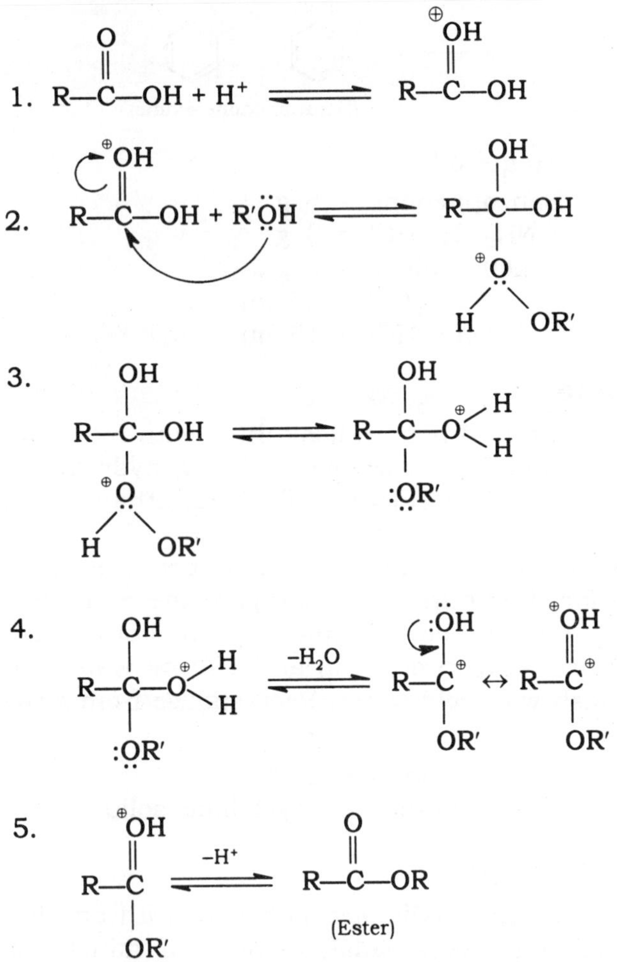

Step 1 is the protonation of the carbonyl group.

Step 2 is the attack of the nucleophile on carbonyl carbon.

Step 3 is the transfer of the proton to one of the OH group.

Step 4 OH group leaves as H_2O molecules.

Step 5 the resonance stabilised protonated ester by loss of proton.

Experiment

Aim: To prepare methyl benzoate from benzoic acid and methanol (Esterification).

Theory: Esterification of benzoic acid and methanol is carried out in the presence of concentrated H_2SO_4. The following reaction takes place.

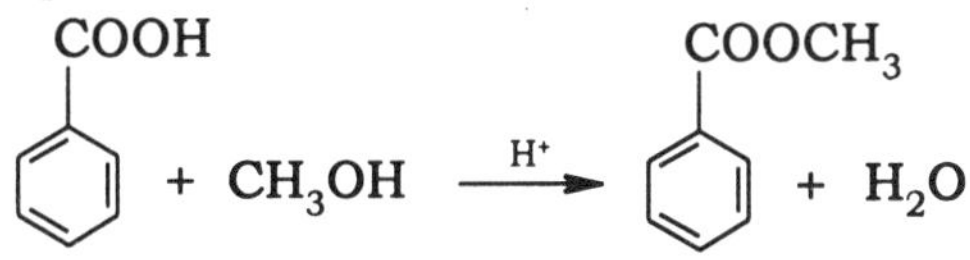

(Benzoic acid) (Methanol) (Methyl benzoate)

Chemicals Required

Benzoic acid = 10 g
Methanol = 30 ml.
Conc. H_2SO_4 = 1 ml.
Ether = 50 ml.

Procedure

In a 250 ml. round bottom flask mix 10 g benzoic acid and 30 ml methanol. Add 1 ml concentrated H_2SO_4 and a few pieces of broken porcelain to prevent bumping. Attach a water condenser and reflux the reaction mixture for one hour on a steam bath. Coal and transfer the solution to a separating funnel. Extract twice with 25 ml portions of ether. Wash the combined ethereal solution with 30 ml water followed by washing with 5% $NaHCO_3$ until no more reaction is observed. Finally wash with water. Dry the solution over Na_2SO_4, and filter. Remove ether on a water bath. Distil the residue using an air condenser. Collect the distillate boiling at 198-200°C.

Yield : 9 g
ppt. : 198°C
Appearance : Colourless liquid

HYDROLYSIS

Experiment

Aim: To prepare p-Bromo aniline from p-Bromo acetanilide (Hydrolysis).

Theory: Anilides on hydrolysis give the corresponding amino compounds. p-Bromo-acetanilide on hydrolysis gives p-Bromo aniline, which is difficult to obtain by the direct bromination of aniline.

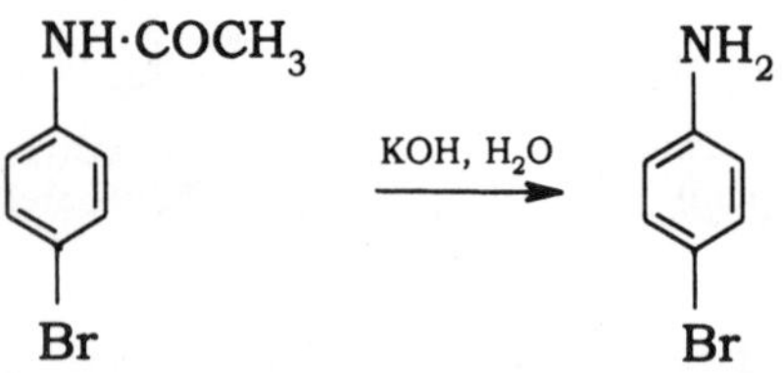

(p-bromo acetanilide) (p-bromoaniline)

Chemicals Required

p-Bromo acetanilide : 7 g
Potassium hydroxide : 4 g
Ethanol : 25 ml.
Ice cold water

Procedure

In a 250 ml round bottom flask fitted with water condenser, mix 7 g of p-bromo acetanilide, 25 ml ethanol, Heat the mixture to get a clear solution. Add 4 g of KOH dissolved in 15 ml water. Boil the reaction mixture for about 30 minutes. Pour the contents in 400 ml beaker containing 50 ml water. Concentrate the contents to about half of its volume on a water bath.

Cool the contents. Pour it in about 50 ml ice cold water. The separated oily product soon solidifies. Filter it and recrystallise it from alcohol.

Yield : 5 g
m.p. : 66°C
Appearance : White crystals

EXPERIMENT

Aim: To prepare p-nitroaniline from p-nitro acetanilide (Hydrolysis).

Theory: Anilides on hydrolysis give the corresponding amino compounds. p-nitro acetanilide on hydrolysis give p-nitroaniline.

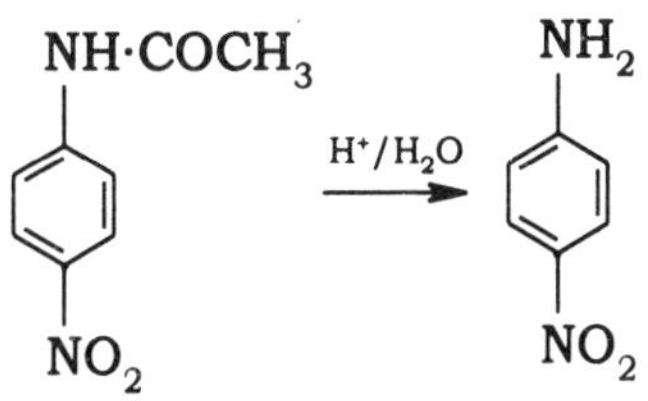

Chemicals Required

p-nitro acetanilide : 3 g
70% H_2SO_4 solution : 15 ml
10% NaOH : 60 ml

Procedure

In a 250 ml round bottom flask, mix 2.5 g p-nitro acetanilide and 15 ml of 70% H_2SO_4. Reflux the reaction mixture for 30 minutes. Cool it and pour the reaction mixture into 400 ml beaker containing 200 ml cold water. Neutralise the reaction mixture with 10% NaOH solution. Filter it and wash with cold water. Recrystallise from hot water.

Yield : 2 g
m.p. : 148°C
Appearance : Yellow crystalline

DIAZOTISATION

Aromatic amines when treated with nitrous acid in cold mineral acid solution, yield aryldiazonium salts, e.g. aniline reacts with nitrous acid in hydrochloric acid solution at 0-5°C to form a solution of benzenediazonium chloride.

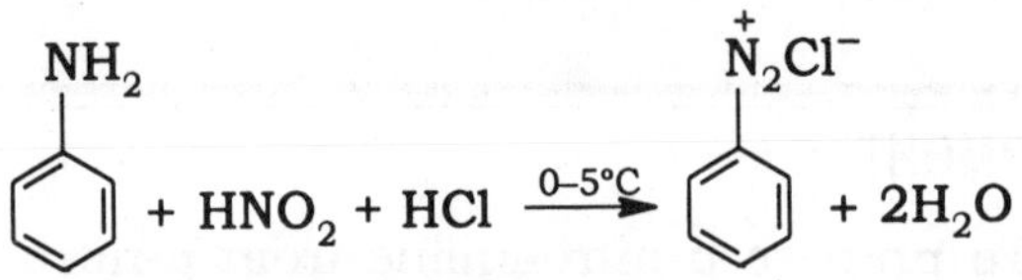

This reaction is called diazotisation reaction. Diazonium salts have the general formula.

$ArN_2^+X^-$

Where $X^- = Cl^-, Br^-, NO_3^-, BF_4^-, HSO_4^-$, etc.

Experiment

Aim: To prepare methyl orange from sulphanilic acid (Diazotisation).

Theory: Methyl orange is prepared by coupling diazotized sulphanilic acid with N, N-dimethylaniline in a weakly acidic solution.

Step 1. Preparation of sodium salt of sulphanilic acid.

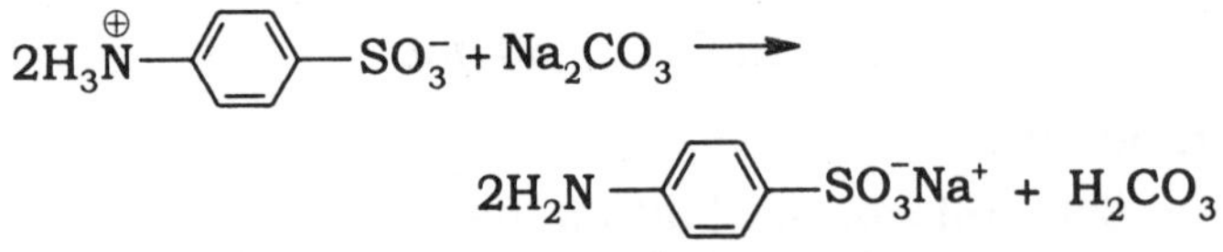

Step 2. Diazotisation step, in which the amino group of sodium salt of sulphanilic acid undergoes normal diazotisation, giving the diazonium-chloride (A).

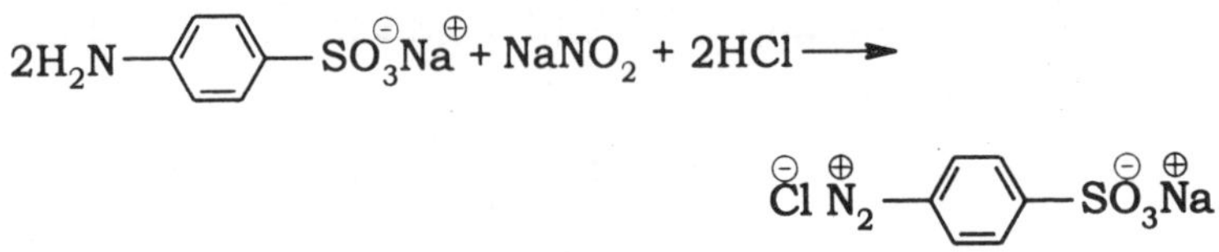

(A)

Step 3. Coupling reaction, when dimethylaniline is added to the diazonium chloride (A) solution, coupling between the diazonium salt and the tertiary amine takes place with the formation of methyl-orange.

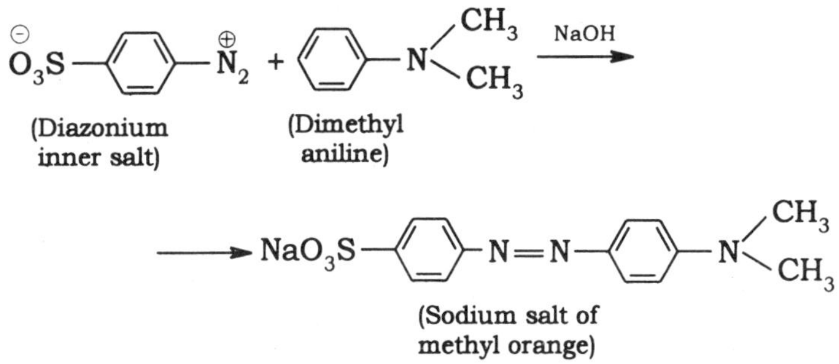

Chemicals Required

(i)	Sulphanilic acid	5 g
(ii)	Sodium carbonate solution (5%)	40 ml
(iii)	Sodium nitrite solution (20%)	10 ml
(iv)	Conc. HCl	6 ml
(v)	Dimethylaniline	3 ml
(vi)	Glacial acetic acid	2 ml
(vii)	Sodium hydroxide solution (20%)	20 ml
(viii)	Sodium chloride	5 g

Procedure

Diazotization step

Dissolve 5 g sulphanilic acid in 40 ml of 5% sodium carbonate. Cool it to O°C by using ice bath. Add slowly cooled 10 ml solution of sodium nitrite with stirring. Add 6 ml conc. HCl solution slowly and a few lumps of crushed ice. Wait for 15 minutes (Test the presence of free nitrous acid by starch iodide paper and if a blue colour develops on the paper by a drop of reaction mixture destroy excess nitrous acid by adding a pinch of solid urea). Crystals of diazobenzene sulphonate separates on cooling. Do not filter these crystals.

Coupling step: In a test tube dissolve 3 ml dimethylaniline in 2 ml glacial acetic acid. Add this solution to the above reaction mixture with constant stirring. Wait for 10 minutes, when crystals of methyl orange starts separating. Add 20 ml of 20% NaOH solution slowly and with constant constant stirring. Add 5 g solid NaCl and warm the reaction mixture on a water bath to dissolve all the NaCl. Cool it in ice bath for 30 minutes. Filter the orange crystals of methyl orange. Dry it in oven at 100°C.

Yield : 6.5 g
m.p. : Not well defined melting point.
Appearance : Deep reddish orange crystals

ELECTROPHILIC AROMATIC SUBSTITUTION REACTIONS

General mechanism of electrophilic aromatic substitution reactions follows the pathways.

Step 1. Generation of electrophiles

$$\text{E—Nu} \rightleftharpoons \text{E}^+ + \text{Nu}^- \quad \text{(Spontaneous dissociation)}$$

E stands for electrophile.
Nu stands for nucleophile.

$$\text{E—Nu} + \underset{\text{Lewis acid}}{\text{A}} \overset{\text{or}}{\rightleftharpoons} \text{E—}\overset{+}{\text{Nu}}\text{—}\overset{-}{\text{A}} \rightleftharpoons \underset{\text{Acid-catalysed dissociation}}{\text{E}^+ + \text{Nu—}\overset{-}{\text{A}}}$$

Step 2. Formation of a resonance stabilised carbonium ion produced by the attack of the electrophile on the benzene ring.

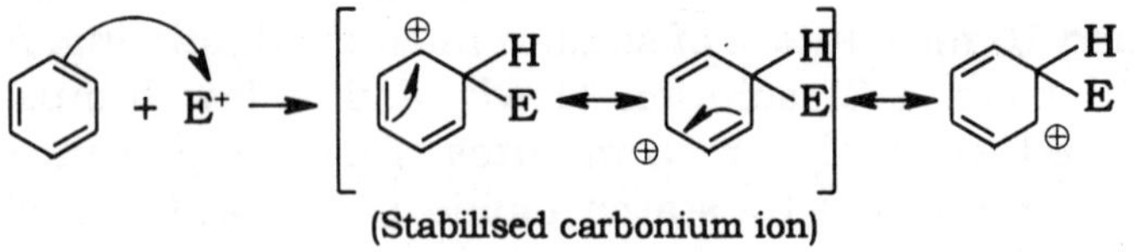

(Stabilised carbonium ion)

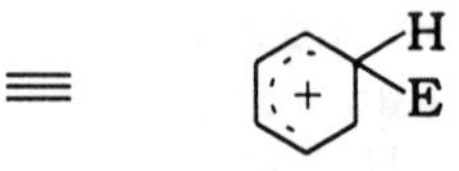

(Resonance hybrid)
or
(σ-complex)

Step 3. Elimination of the proton from the stabilised carbonium ion by a base (say : B^-) to yield the final substitution product.

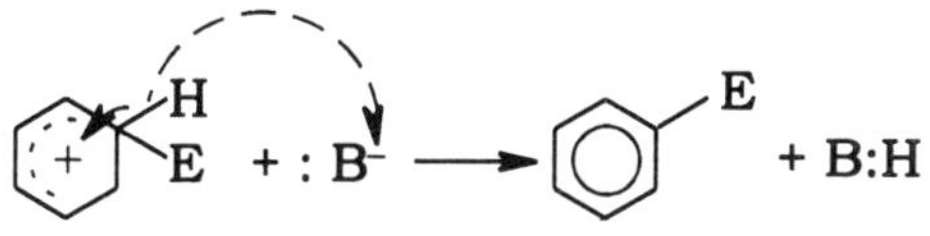

(σ-complex) (Substitution product)

Following are the examples of electrophilic aromatic substitution reactions.

(i) Halogenation

Benzene reacts with chlorine or bromine in the presence of a Lewis catalyst such as $AlCl_3$, $FeCl_3$, $FeBr_3$ when substitution in the ring takes place, a proton being lost as HCl or HBr.

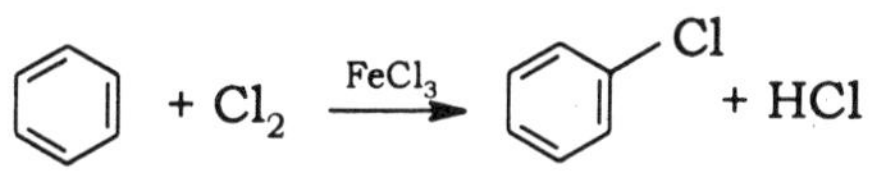

(Benzene) (Chlorobenzone)

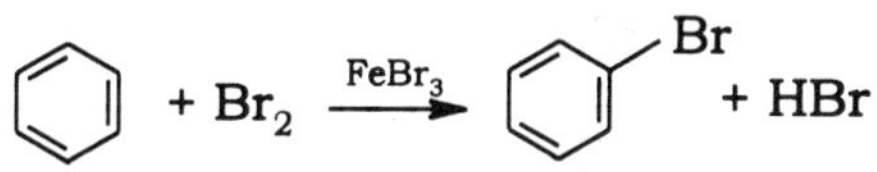

(Benzene) (Bromobenzone)

Mechanism

Step 1. Generation of the electrophile Br^+ or Cl^+

$$Cl{-}Cl + FeCl_3 \longrightarrow Cl^{\oplus} + FeCl_4^{\ominus}$$

Step 2. Formation of a resonance-stabilised carbonium ion or σ-complex.

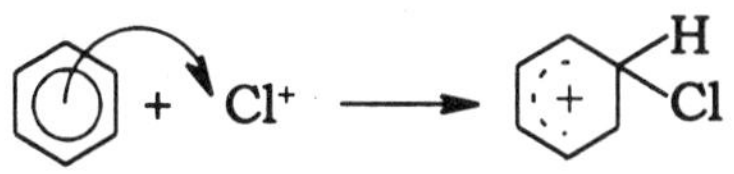

(σ-complex)

Step 3. Elimination of a proton.

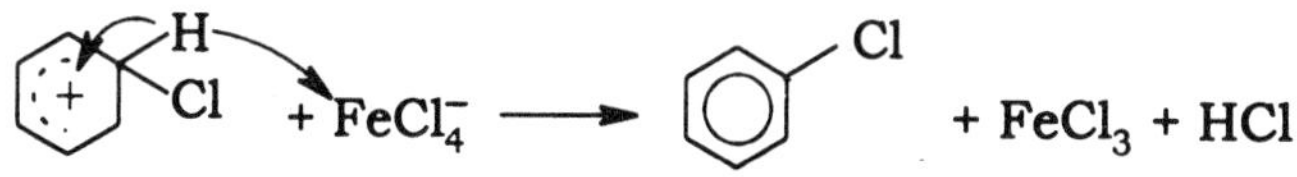

(σ-complex) (Chlorobenzene)

(ii) Nitration

Benzene reacts with nitric acid in presence of sulphuric acid to form nitrobenzene.

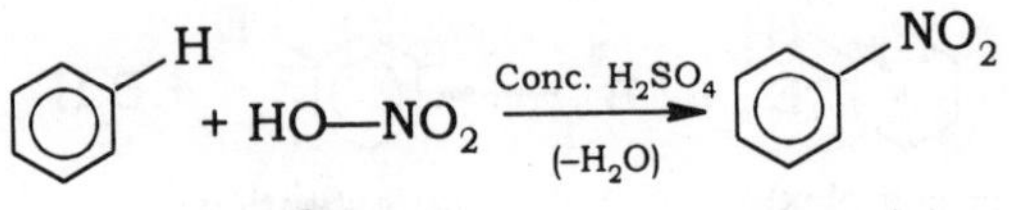

Mechanism

Step 1. Generation of the electrophile nitronium ion by the protonation of concentrated sulphuric acid.

$$H_2SO_4 + HNO_3 \longrightarrow HSO_4^{\ominus} + H_2NO_3^{\oplus}$$

$$H_2NO_3^{\oplus} + H_2SO_4 \longrightarrow HSO_4^{\ominus} + H_3O^{\oplus} + NO_2^{\oplus}$$

(Nitronium ion)

Step 2. Formation of σ-complex or stable resonance hybrid.

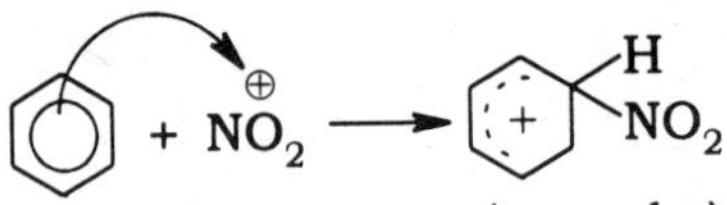

(σ-complex)

Step 3. Elimination of proton from σ-complex.

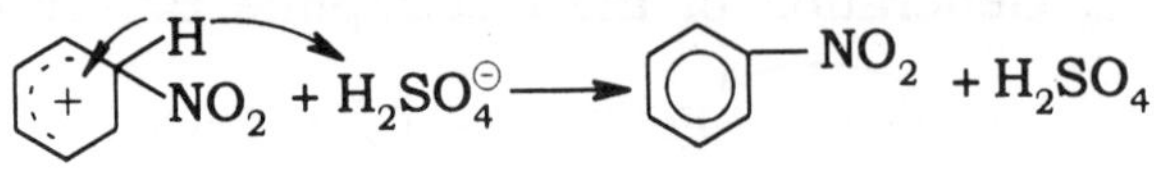

(iii) Sulphonation

Benzene may be sulphonated by treating it with concentrated sulphuric acid and gives benzene sulphonic acid.

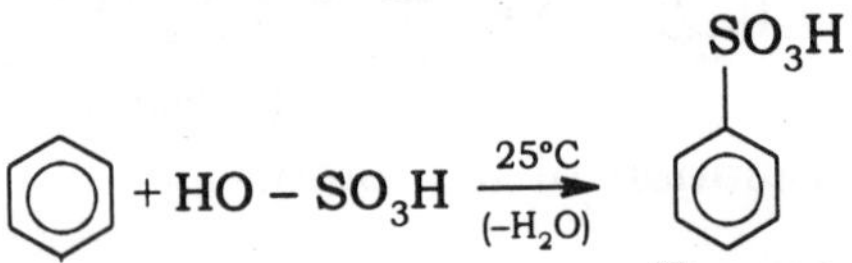

(Benzene sulphonic acid)

Mechanism

Step 1. Generation of electrophile.

$$2H_2SO_4 \rightleftharpoons H_3\overset{\oplus}{O} + HS\overset{\ominus}{O}_4 + SO_3$$

Although SO_3 is a neutral molecule, its sulphur atom carries positive charge due to resonance of the molecule.

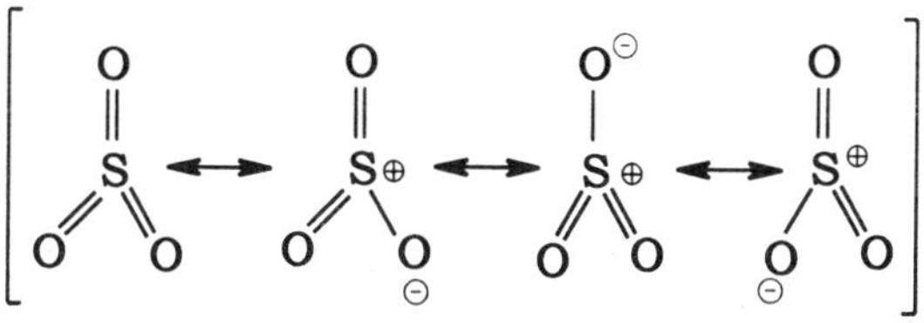

Therefore SO_3 acts as a electrophile.

Step 2. Formation of σ-complex.

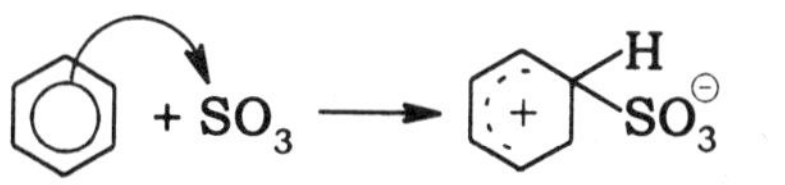

(σ-complex)

Step 3. Elimination of a proton

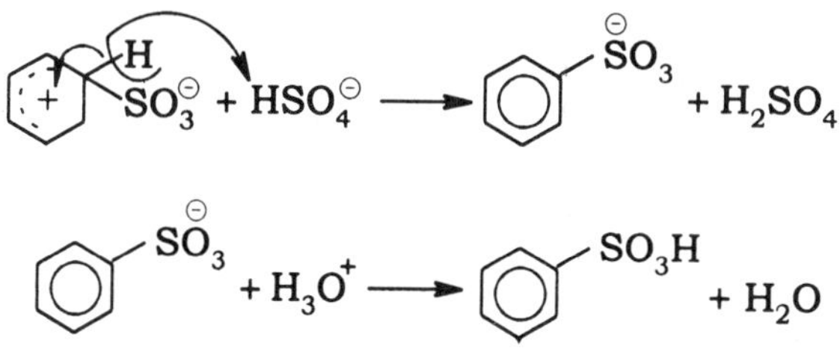

(Benzene sulphonic acid)

(IV) Friedel-Crafts Reactions

Friedel crafts reaction are of two general types

(a) Friedel-Crafts Alkylation.

(b) Friedel-Crafts Acylation.

(a) Friedel-Crafts Alkylation

This reaction involves the introduction of an alkyl group in the benzene ring, e.g. benzene reacts with an alkyl halide (RCl or RBr) in the presence of anhydrous $AlCl_3$ as catalyst:

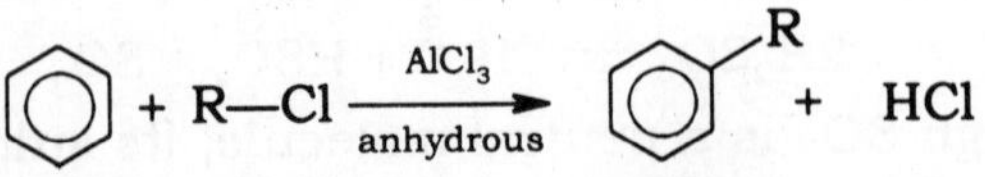

(Alkyl benzene)

The alkylating agent used in Friedel-Crafts alkylation is an alkyl halide. The catalyst is a Lewis acid $AlCl_3$, BF_3, $FeCl_3$, etc.

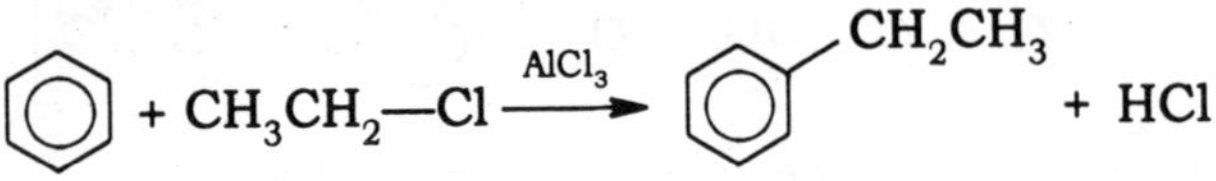

(Ethyl benzene)

Mechanism

Step 1. Generation of electrophile.

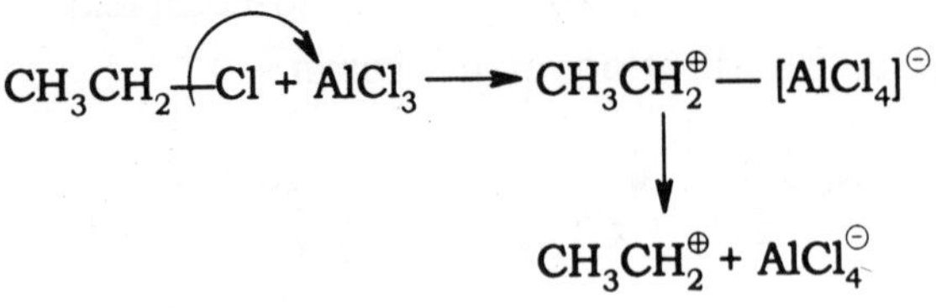

Step 2. Formation of the σ-complex.

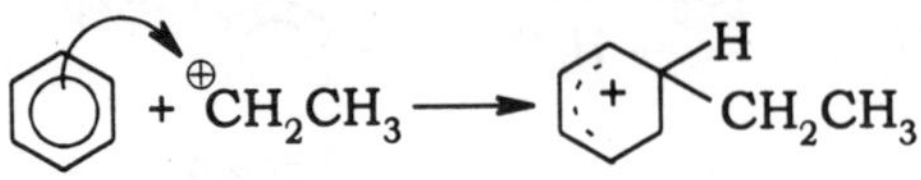

σ-complex

Step 3. Elimination of proton from σ-complex.

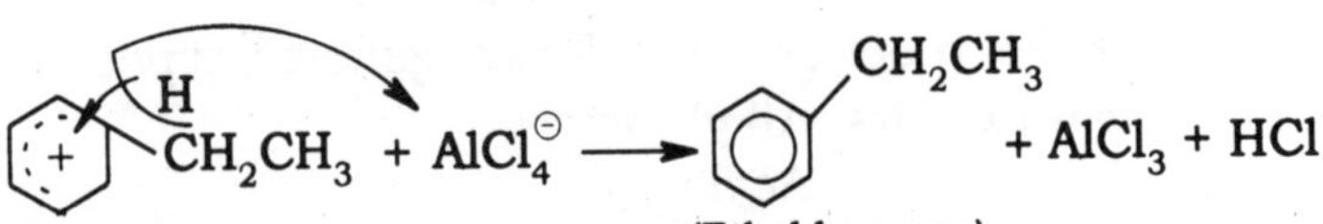

(Ethyl benzene)

(b) Friedel-Crafts Acylation

This reaction involves, the introduction of an acyl group (RCO—) in the aromatic ring in the presence of anlydrous

$AlCl_3$ (or other Lewis acids like BF_3, $FeCl_3$, $ZnCl_2$ etc.) The acylating agents employed are acid chlorides, acid anhydrides and esters.

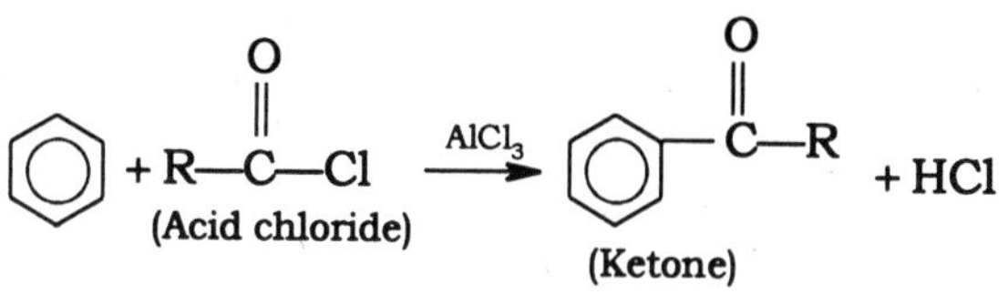

e.g.

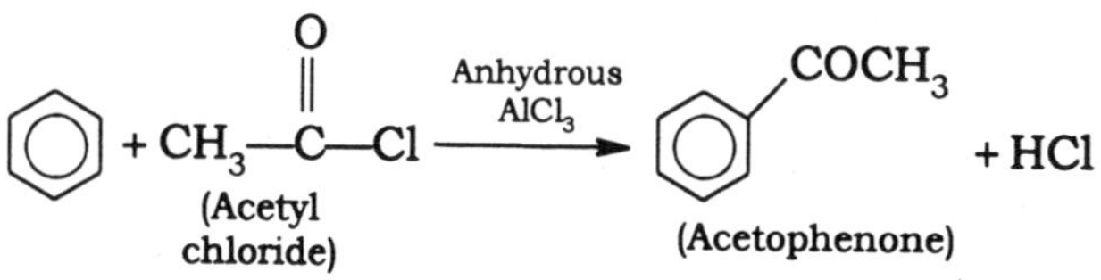

Mechanism

Step 1. Generation of electrophile.

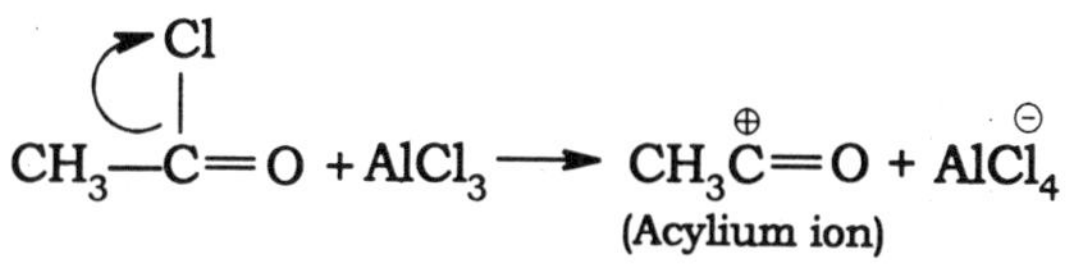

Step 2. Formation of σ-Complex.

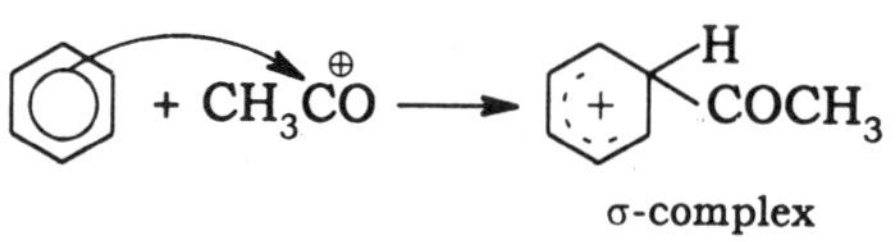

Step 3. Elimination of proton.

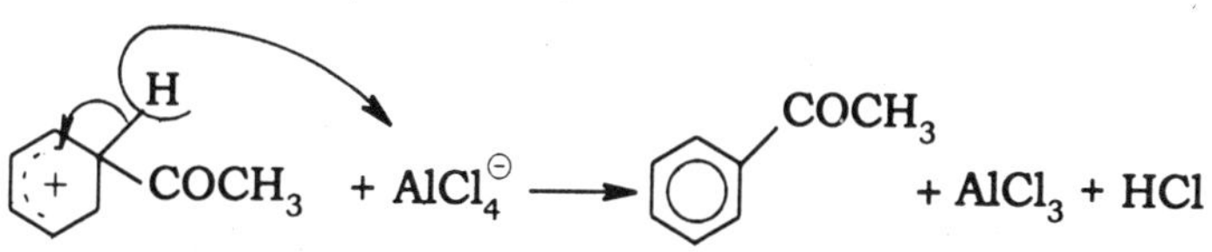

Experiment

Aim: To prepare p-Bromo acetanilide from acetanilide (bromination).

Theory: Acetanilide on bromination gives a mixture of o- and p-bromo acetanilide. The ortho compound is formed in only small amount, however, and being more soluble in ethanol than the para compound can be readily eliminated by recrystallisation.

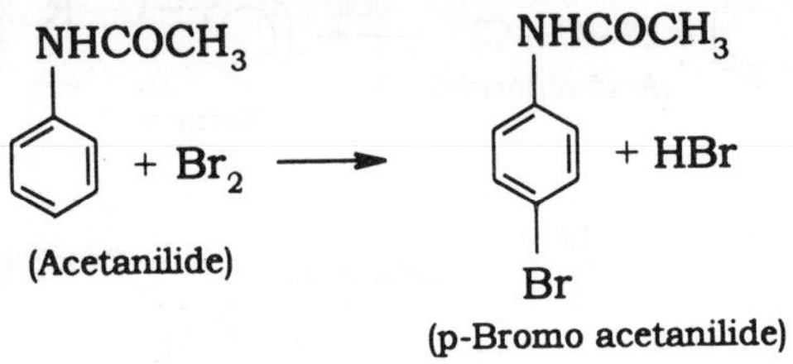

Chemicals Required

Acetanilide	:	2 g
Glacial acetic acid	:	20 ml
Liquid bromine	:	1 ml

Procedure

Dissolve 2 g of powdered acetanilide in 8 ml glacial acetic acid in a 100 ml conical flask.

In another flask prepare a bromine solution by adding 1 ml of liquid bromine in 12 ml of glacial acetic acid.

Add this solution very slowly to the acetanilide solution with constant stirring.

Pour the reaction mixture intro 100 ml of cold water. Filter the ppts. Recrystallize from rectified spirit.

Yield	:	2g
m.p.	:	167°C
Appearance	:	Colourless crystals

Experiment

Aim: To prepare nitrobenzene from benzene (Nitration).

Theory: Aromatic compounds on treatment with nitric acid or mixture of nitric acid and sulphuric acid give nitroderivatives. The reaction is known as nitration.

nitric acid first produces nitronium ion ($\overset{\oplus}{NO_2}$). Then it attacks the nucleus to from σ-complex or stabilised carbonium ion. σ-complex loses proton and produce the nitro-derivatives.

$$HNO_3 + 2H_2SO_4 \longrightarrow \overset{\oplus}{NO_2} + H_3\overset{\oplus}{O} + 2HSO_4^-$$

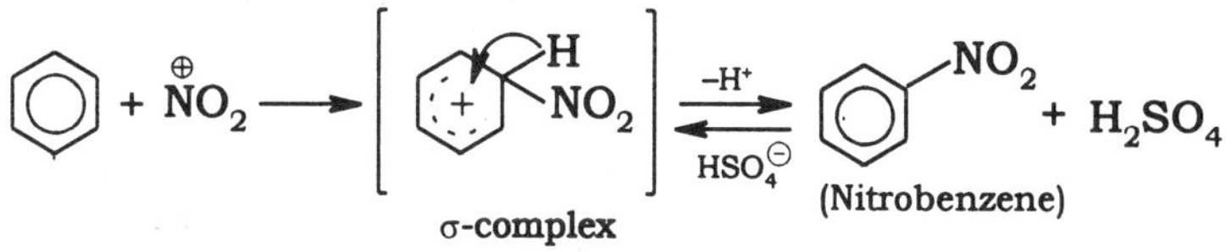

Chemicals Required

(i) Benzene 10 ml
(ii) Conc. HNO_3 12 ml
(iii) Conc. H_2SO_4 14 ml
(iv) Ice

Procedure

In a 250 ml round bottom flask, take 12 ml conc. HNO_3 and add 14 ml conc. H_2SO_4 slowly, with shaking and cooling. Add 10 ml benzene drop by drop with vigorous shaking. The temp. should not be allowed to exceed 50°C. Heat the reaction mixture on a water bath at 50-60°C for 20 minutes. Cool and pour on 200 ml ice cold water. Stir and transfer it in a separating funnel and separate the lower layer of nitrobenzene.

Yield : 10 g
Boiling point : 210°C
Appearance : Pale yellow liquid

Experiment

Aim: To prepare m-dinitrobenzene from nitrobenzene (Nitration).

Theory: Nitrobenzene reacts with fuming nitric acid in the presence of concentrated sulphuric acid and gives m-dinitrobenzene.

Step 1. Generation of electrophile.

$$HNO_3 + 2\,H_2SO_4 \longrightarrow \overset{\oplus}{N}O_2 + \overset{\oplus}{H_3}O + 2HSO_4^{\ominus}$$

Step 2. Formation of σ-complex.

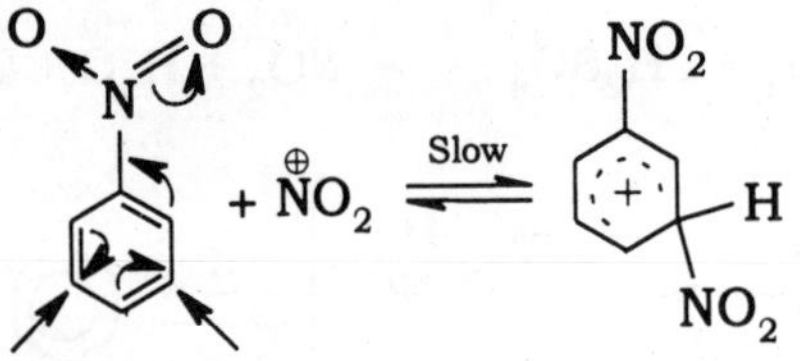

Step 3. Elimination of proton.

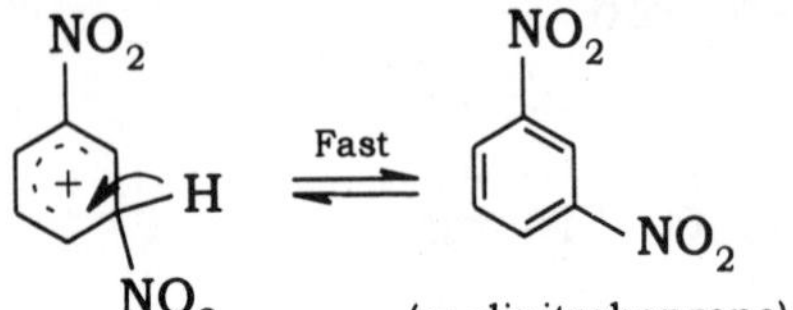

(m-dinitrobenzene)

Chemicals Required

Nitrobenzene	:	9 ml
Fuming nitric acid	:	10 ml
Concentrated H_2SO_4	:	12 ml
Ice cold water		
Ice		

Procedure

In a 250 ml round bottom flask take 9 ml fuming nitric acid and add 12 ml conc. sulphuric acid slowly with shaking and cooling. With vigorous shaking add 9 ml of nitrobenzene in fractions. On addition of nitrobenzene, heat is evolved and the colour of the mixture becomes dark. Fit an air condenser and heat the flask on a water bath till a few drops of the reaction mixture gives a precipitate when added to small quantity of cold water (after about 30 minutes). Cool the reaction mixture and pour with vigorous shaking into 200 ml cold water containing a few pieces of ice. Filter the yellow solid and crystallise from alcohol.

Yield : 9 g
Melting point : 90°C
Appearance : Pale yellow crystals

Experiment

Aim: To prepare picric acid from phenol (Nitration).

Theory: Phenol can be easily nitrated with the help of nitric acid and sulphuric acid. The reaction is very vigorous and sometimes violent.

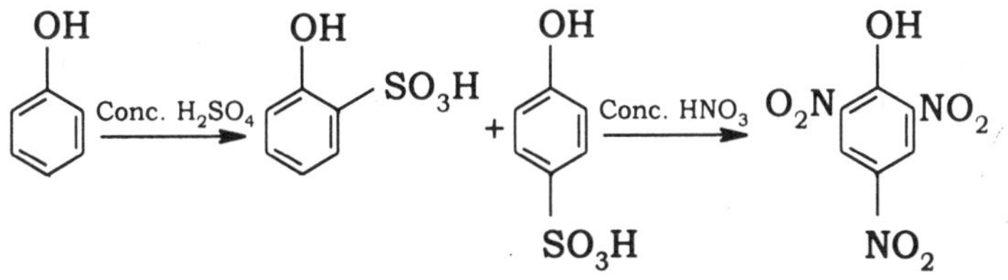

(Picric acid)

Phenol is largely destroyed by oxidation if the phenol is directly treated with a mixture of nitric acid and sulphuric acid. A more convenient procedure for obtaining picric acid from phenol is first to sulphonate the phenol and then to nitrate the sulphonated products with concentrated nitric acid.

Chemicals Required

(i) Phenol 5 g
(ii) Conc. H_2SO_4 6 ml
(iii) Conc. HNO_3 19 ml

Procedure

Dissolve 5 g phenol in 6 ml conc. H_2SO_4 in a 250 ml conical flask. Shake, heat on a water bath for 30 minutes, cool and add 19 ml of conc. HNO_3 to it dropwise with shaking. Brown fumes are evolved. When the reaction subsides, heat the flask on a water bath for one hour with occasional shaking. Cool and add 50 ml ice cold water. Crystals of picric acid appear. Filter and wash with water. Recrystallize from alcohol.

Yield : 8 g
m.p. : 122°C
Appearance : Pale yellow

Experiment

Aim: To prepare sulphanilic acid from aniline (sulphonation).

Theory: Aniline when heated with concentrated H_2SO_4 forms anilinium hydrogen sulphate, which eliminate a water molecule to form phenyl sulphamic acid. Phenyl sulphamic acid on heating rearranages to sulphanilic acid.

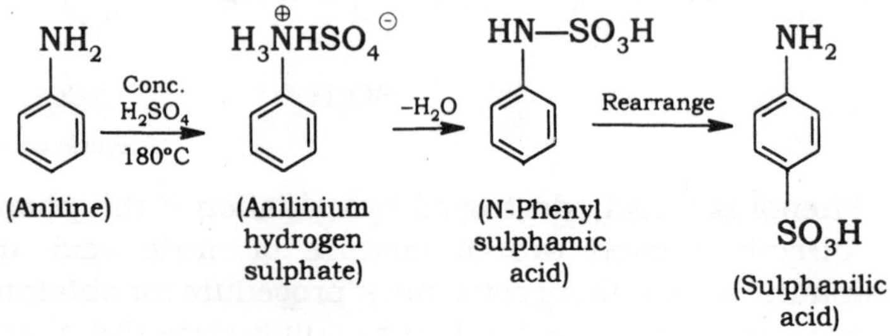

Chemicals Required

Aniline : 5 ml
Conc. H_2SO_4 : 10 ml

Procedure

In a 250 ml round bottom flask take 5 ml aniline and add 10 ml conc. H_2SO_4 in small portions with stirring and cooling the flask in an ice bath. After the addition of sulphuric acid, heat the flask in an oil bath at 180°C in a fume cupboard for about five hours. Cool the flask and pour the contents very carefully and slowly with stirring into 1/2 kg of crushed ice taken in a beaker. Filter it and wash it with cold water. Recrystallise from boiling water.

Yield : 5g
m.p. : No well defined melting point
Appearance : White shining crystals.

Experiment

Aim: To prepare o-Benzoyl benzoic acid from phthalic anhydride (Friedel-Crafts Reaction).

Theory: This preparation is an example of Friedel Crafts acylation reaction, which utilizes aluminium chloride as catalyst and forms acyl carbonium ion. Mechanism of the reaction is as follows:

Step 1. Formation of Acyl carbonium ion.

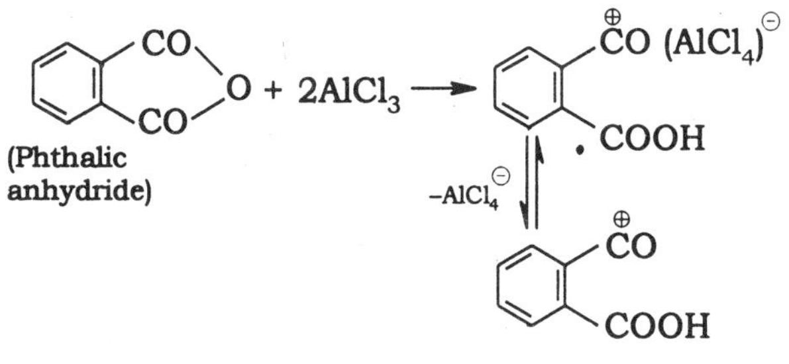

(Acyl carbonium ion)

Step 2. Reaction of benzene with acyl carbonium ion.

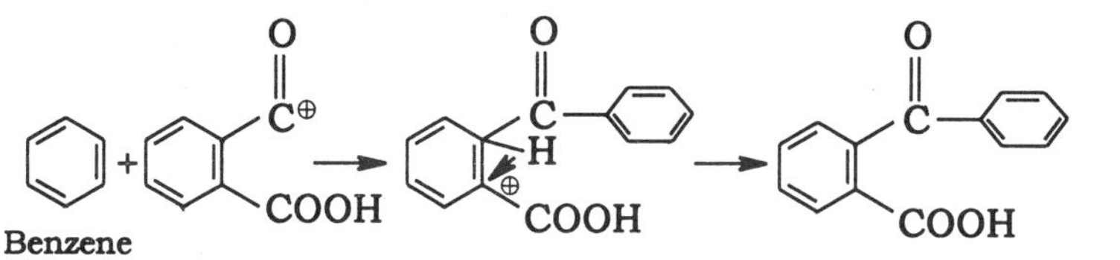

(O-Benzoyl benzoic acid)

Chemicals Required

Phthalic anhydride	:	5 g
Benzene	:	50 ml
Anhydrous $AlCl_3$	:	10 g
Conc. HCl	:	10 ml
10% Na_2CO_3 solution	:	40 ml

Procedure

In a 250 ml round bottom flask mix 5 g phthalic anhydride, 25 ml benzene and 10 g anhydrous $AlCl_3$.

Shake vigorously for half an hour. The reaction will start with the evolution of HCl gas. Heat the reaction mixture on a boiling water bath for an hour. Cool the flask and add 50 g crushed ice and shake. Add conc. HCl till a clear solution is obtained. Distill excess of benzene and cool the residue in ice bath.

Filter it and dissolve the solid in 40 ml of 10% Na_2CO_3 solution and filter again to remove any suspended particles. Acidify the filtrate with conc. HCl stirring with a glass rod. The acid separates out as a solid. Filter and dry in air.

Yield : 4 g
m.p. : 120°C
Appearance : Colourless crystals

Experiment

Aim: To prepare triphenyl methane from Benzene and Chloroform (Friedel-Crafts reaction).

Theory: This preparation is an example of Friedel Craft alkylation reaction, which utilizes $AlCl_3$ as catalyst and forms alkyl carbonium ion.

Step 1. Formation of carbonium ion.

$$\underset{\text{(Chloroform)}}{CHCl_3} + AlCl_3 \rightleftharpoons [AlCl_4]^{\ominus} + \overset{\oplus}{C}HCl_2$$

Step 2. Formation of σ-complex.

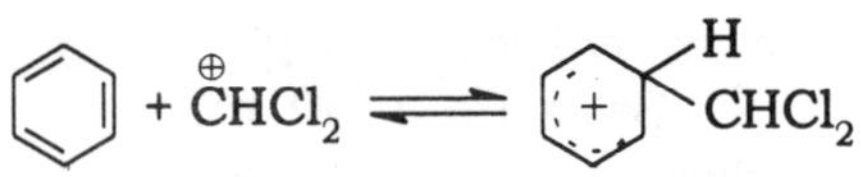

Step 3. Elimination of proton.

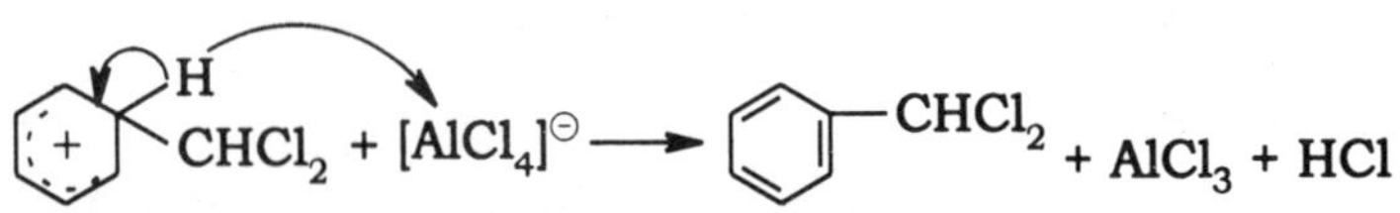

Step 4.

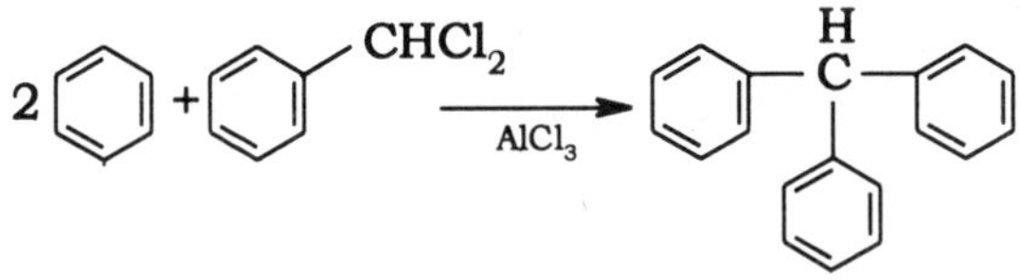

(Triphenyl-methane)

Chemicals Required

Benzene	:	50 ml
Chloroform	:	6 ml
Anhydrous $AlCl_3$	:	7 g

Procedure

In a 250 ml round bottom flask fitted with a reflux water condenser mix 50 ml dry benzene and 6 ml dry chloroform, Add 7 g of powdered aluminimum chloride in small fractions. Shake the reaction mixture and boil on a sand bath for half an hour. Cool and pour into 50 ml cold water.Distill the excess benzene by heating on a water bath. Now distill the remaining fraction, first an oil will distill over and then an orange coloured viscous liquid will pass over, which will solidify in the receiver. Recrystallise the solid product from hot alcohol.

Yield	:	5 g
m.p.	:	92°C
Appearance	:	Colourless plates

Rearrangement reactions

Rearrangement reactions are those reactions which proceed by a rearrangement or reshuffling of the atoms or groups in the molecule to produce a structural isomer of the original substance. These reactions may proceed either by an intramolecular rearrangement or inter-molecular rearrangement.

(I) Intramolecular rearrangements

Examples of intramolecular change are given below:

(a) *Isomerization:* Butane changes to isobutane

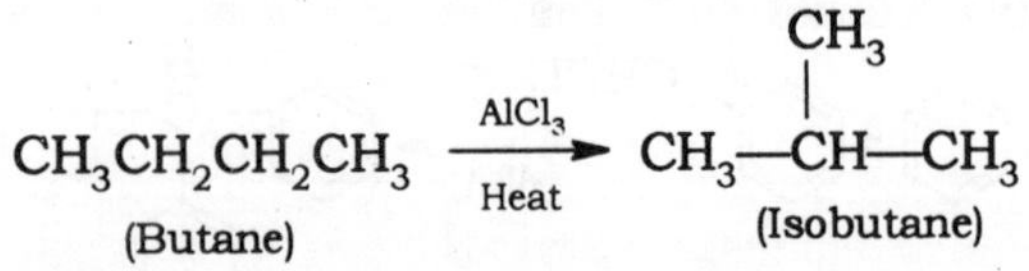

(b) *Beckmann rearrangement:* When a ketoxime is treated with acidic catalyst such as H_2SO_4, PCl_5, etc. it gets converted into a substituted amide.

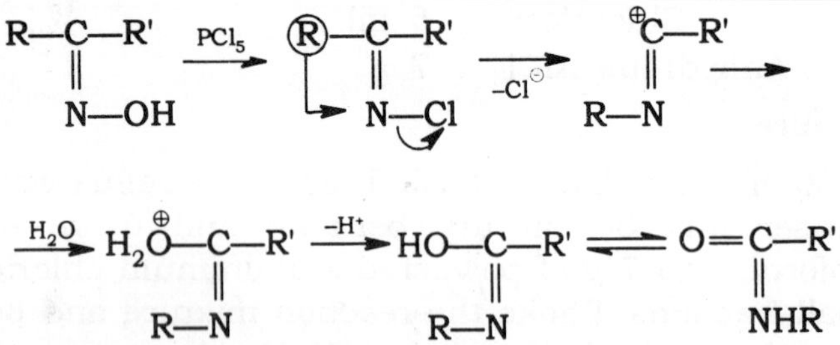

(c) *Benzidine rearrangements:* On warming hydrazobenzene with mineral acids, benzidine is formed.

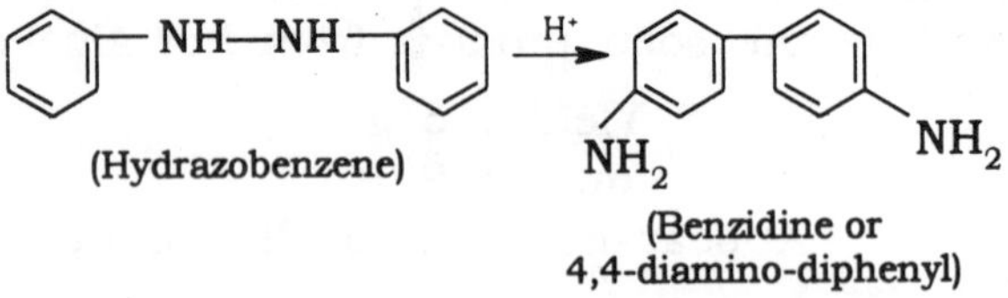

(II) Intermolecular rearrangements

In these rearrangements, the atom or group undergoing migration becomes completely free from the rest of the molecule and later on gets reattached at some site of the rest of the molecule producing thereby structural isomer of the original substance. Examples of this type of rearrangements are:

(a) *Orton rearrangement:* In this rearrangement, N-Chloroacetanilide gets converted into a mixture of o- and p-Chloroacetanilide on treatment with dil HCl.

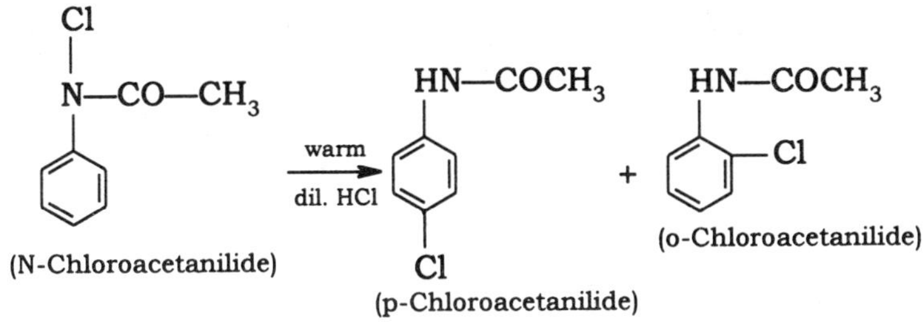

(b) *Diazoaminobenzene rearrangement:* Diazoaminobenzene in weakly acidic media rearranges to p-aminoazobenzene.

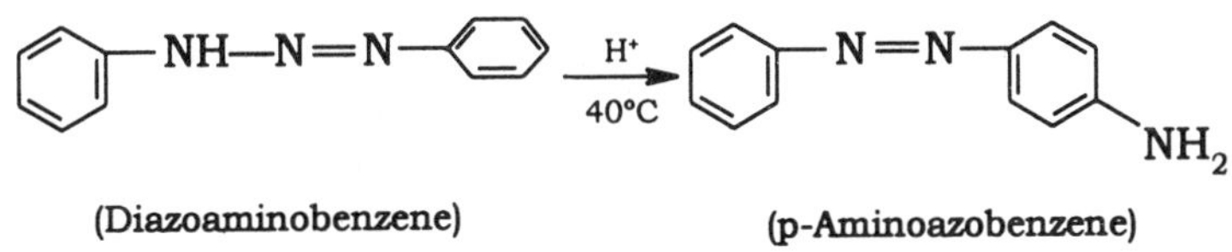

Experiment

Aim: To prepare benzanilide from benzophenone oxime (Beckmann rearrangement)

Theory: Keto oximes in presence of certain acidic reagents such as sulphuric acid, PCl_5, thionyl chloride, undergo molecular rearrangement to form N-substituted acid amides. The mechanism of the above preparation is as follows:

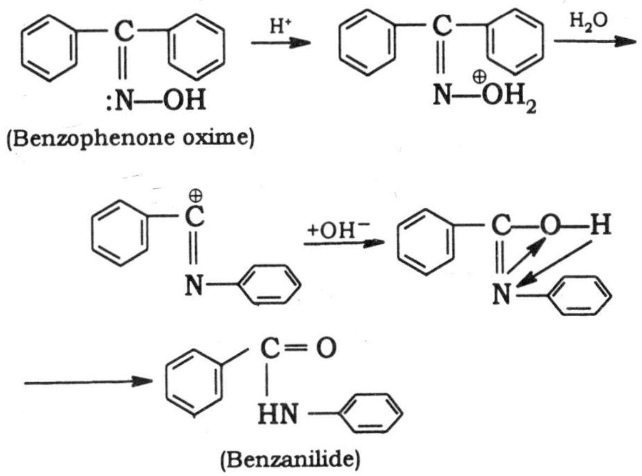

Chemicals Required

Benzophenone oxime	: 4 g
PCl_5	: 10 g
	or
$SOCl_2$ (Thionyl chloride)	: 7 ml.
Ether	: 50 ml

Procedure

In 250 ml conical flask mix 4 g benzophenone oxime and 50 ml dry ether. Shake (or warm if necessary) to get a clear solution. Add 10 g PCl_5 (or 7 ml $SOCl_2$). Shake well for five minutes. Distill off ether on a water bath. Cool and add 40 ml water. Boil for half an hour and cool again. Decant the supernatent liquid and recrystallise the product left in the flask from hot alcohol.

Yield	: 3 g
m.p.	: 162°C
Appearance	: White crystalline solid

Experiment

Aim: To prepare benzilic acid from benzil. (Benzilic acid rearrangement).

Theory: α-Aromatic diketones on treatment with alcoholic alkalies rearrange to form α -hydroxy acids. Benzil thus gives benzilic acid. The probable mechanism of this reaction is:

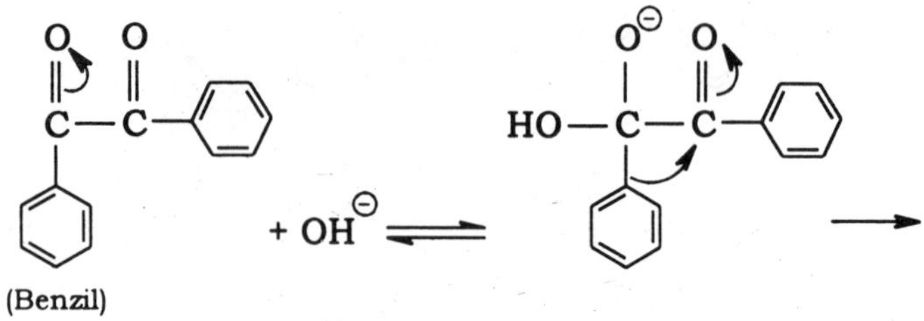

(Benzil)

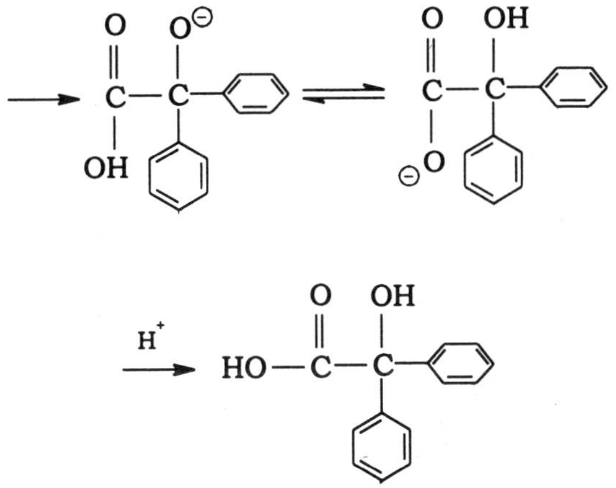

(Benzilic acid)

Chemicals Required

Benzil	:	5 g
Potassium hydroxide	:	5 g
Ethanol	:	20 ml
Dilute H_2SO_4		

Procedure

In a 250 ml round bottom flask mix 5 g benzil, 20 ml ethanol and 10 ml of 50% aq. solution of potassium hydroxide. Shake well to get purple colour or bluish-black solution. Boil the reaction mixture for about 20 minutes on a water bath using reflux water condenser. Cool and transfer the reaction mixture in a china dish. Cool it in an ice bath. The potassium salt of benzilic acid separates out, filter it and wash throughly with cold water. Dissolve the salt in 30 ml water and acidify the solution with concentrated HCl with constant stirring. A red brown precipitate of the acid is formed. Filter and wash it with cold water.

Recrystallise from benzene (about 30 ml) using activated charcoal. Filter the boiling solution through pre-heated funnel. Benzilic acid readily crystallises as the solution cools (Alternatively recrystallise from much hot water)

Yield : 4 g
m.p. : 150°C
Appearance : Colourless shining crystals

Experiment

Aim: To prepare 2,5-Dihydroxy acetophenone from hydroquinone diacetate (Fries-rearrangement).

Theory: Esters of phenolic compounds on treatment with anhydrous aluminium chloride yield o- and p- (or both) hydroxy-ketones. This reaction is reffered to as Fries-rearrangement. It is believed to occur by first cleavage of the ester to produce an acylium ($R\overset{\oplus}{C}O$) ion, which then reacts with the electron rich o- and p-positions of the phenolic compound in the usual Friedel Crafts type reactions.

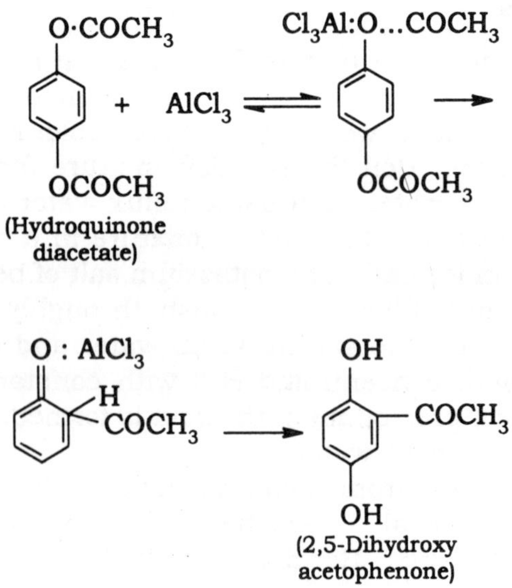

Chemicals Required

Hydroquinone diacetate : 10 g
Anhydrous aluminium chloride : 20 g
Conc. HCl : 7 ml
Crushed Ice

Procedure

In a 250 ml round bottom flask, mix 10 g powdered hydroquinone diacetate and 20 g anhydrous $AlCl_3$. Attach an air condenser and heat the flask between 115-120°C in an oil bath in the fume chamber for half an hour. When the evolution of HCl gas starts, raise the temperature to 160-165°C and continue heating for about one hour. Cool the reaction mixture, add about 50 g crushed ice and 7 ml conc. HCl and swirl. Filter it and wash with ice cold water. Recrystallise from aqueous alcohol.

Yield : 4 g
m.p. : 202°C
Appearance : Colourless crystals

MISCELLANEOUS REACTIONS

Experiment

Aim: To prepare phenolphthalein from phenol and phthalic anhydride.

Theory: Phenolphthalein is prepared by condensing two molecules of phenol with phthalic anhydride (one molecule)

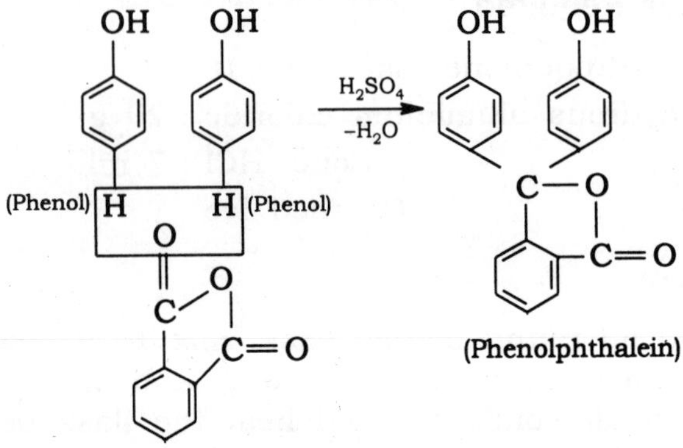

Chemicals Required

(i)	Phenol	12.5 g
(ii)	Phthalic anhydride	6 g
(iii)	Conc. H_2SO_4	4 ml
(iv)	Dil. NaOH solution	
(v)	Dil. acetic acid.	

Procedure

In a 250 ml round bottom flask, mix 12.5 g phenol and 6 g phthalic anhydride. Heat in an oil bath until the mixture of solid melts. Add 4 ml conc. H_2SO_4. Heat the flask in an oil bath at 105°C for 5 hours until the mass becomes semi solid and of a dark red colour. Pour the hot reaction mixture in 300 ml hot water and boil until the odour of phenol has disappeared. Cool and filter the yellow ppt. in minimum amount of dil. NaOH solution. Filter off any residue obtained and acidify the filterate with dilute acetic acid and few drops of dil. HCl. Allow to stand over night. Filter the light yellow crystals. Dissolve it in minimum amount of alcohol and add 2 g animal charcoal. Reflux the solution for half an hour on a water bath. Filter the hot solution and evaporate the filterate on a water bath till pure crystals of phenolphthalein are obtained.

Yield: 4.5 g
m.p. : 256-258°C
Appearance : Colourless crystals

Aim: To isolate caffeine from the tea leaves.

Theory: Caffeine is 1,3,7-trimethyl xanthine. It is an alkaloid present in a tea leaves. Tea leaves contain 1 to 5% caffeine. Caffeine is soluble in water and thus can be extracted by boiling the tea leaves with water.

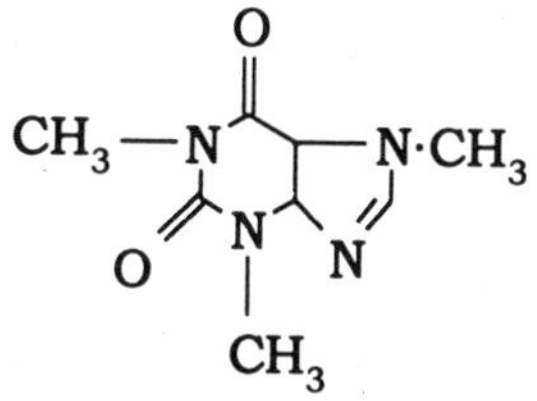

(Caffeine)

Chemicals Required

Tea leaves	=	50 gm
Chloroform	=	100 ml
Lead acetate	=	10% solution
Petroleum	=	50 ml

Procedure

Boil 50 gm dry tea leaves in a 400 ml beaker with 250 ml water for half an hour. Filter it while hot. To the filtrate add 50 ml of 10% lead acetate solution to precipitate tannins (which is a naturally occuring polyphenols). Filter it and concentrate the filtrate on a sand bath to about 25 minutes. Take this filtrate in a separating funnel and extract caffeine from the filtrate by treating it with 25 ml of chloroform four times. Separate and collect the chloroform layer in a distillation flask and distill off the chloroform by heating on a water bath. Cool the residue and add 25 ml of petroleum ether and stir the mixture for 5 minutes. Filter the crude caffeine.

Yield	:	0.5-0.7 gm
m.p.	:	234-236°C
Appearance	:	Colourless needle like crystals

Test for Caffeine

Dissolve 0.1 mg of caffeine in hot water + ($K_4[Fe(CN)_6]$ + HNO_3) $\xrightarrow{\text{warm}}$ Prussian blue colour (Confirms-caffeine)

Aim: To isolate casein and lactose from milk.

Theory: Casein is a phosphoprotein. It contains at least 15 amino acids. Cow milk contains about 3% of casein. It is an amorphous, odourless, tasteless and hygroscopic white solid. It is insoluble in organic solvent but soluble in NaOH solution. The pH of fresh milk is approx. 6.5-6.7, when it is acidified to pH 4.0.-4.5 casein precipitates out. Lactose is a di-saccharides sugar soluble in water. It occurs in the milk of all mammals. It is readily soluble in water.

Chemicals Required

Milk = 200 ml
Acetic acid
NaOH, Ethanol, Ether, Magnesium-carbonate

Procedure

(i) Dilute 200 ml of milk with 300 ml of water and warm at 50°C. Add 10% acetic acid dropwise with constant stirring to precipitate the casein. Filter it and wash it with a mixture of 10 ml water + 40 ml of ethanol + 20 ml ether to remove all the fats. Dry the wet solid.

(ii) *Isolation of lactose:* Take the aqueous filtrate from casein in a 400 ml beaker and boil to precipitate soluble proteins. Filter it. In order to neutralize the filtrate, add 10% aq. solution of magnesium carbonate. Evaporate the filtrate. Extract with ethanol, dissolve the residue in water, filter and concentrate to get a syrup. Keep the syrup in an ice bath, whereby the crystals of lactose separate out.

CHAPTER

7

Qualitative Organic Analysis Viva-Voce

CHAPTER 1

Q.1. What is Lassaigne's test? For which purpose it is used?

Ans. Lassaigne's test is used to detect the presence of nitrogen, sulphur and halogens in an organic compound.

Q.2. Why ignition tube must be dry in fusion test?

Ans. Ignition tube must be dried otherwise, water present in it will react with it and make it inactive.

$$2Na + 2H_2O \rightarrow 2NaOH + H_2 \uparrow$$

Q.3. Why distilled water is used for the preparation of sodium extract?

Ans. Tap water may contain chloride ions which will give positive test for chlorine even in its absence hence, the sodium extract is prepared in distilled water only.

Q.4. Why freshly prepared solution of sodium nitroprusside is used for the detection of sulphur?

Ans. Sodium nitroprusside is unstable in aqueous solution, therefore freshly prepared solution is used.

Q.5. Why aromatic compounds burn with a smoky flame?

Ans. Aromatic compounds have higher percentage of

carbon, which is not fully oxidised and hence, burn with a smoky flame which contains unburnt carbon particles.

Q.6. Define chemically Tollen's reagent?

Ans. Tollen's reagent chemically is ammoniacal silver nitrate solution.

Q.7. What is Fehling's solution?

Ans. Fehling's solution is a mixture of copper sulphate and sodium hydroxide along with the solution of sodium potassium tartrate.

Q.8. Which organic compounds give silver mirror test with Tollen's reagent?

Ans. Organic compounds which are easily oxidisable and are of reducing nature give silver mirror test. Such compounds are aldehydes, reducing sugars such as glucose and fructose, formic acid and hydroquinone.

Q.9. Give the chemistry for the detection of nitrogen, sulphur and halogens by Lassaigne's test.

Ans. The organic compound is fused with sodium metal. This converts nitrogen, sulphur and halogens to sodium cyanide, sodium sulphide and sodium halides respectively, which are soluble in water. Following are the chemical reactions which take place in the identification of these elements :

(i) For detection of nitrogen

$$C + N + Na \rightarrow NaCN$$

$$FeSO_4 + 2NaOH \rightarrow Fe(OH)_2\downarrow + Na_2SO_4$$

$$Fe(OH)_2 + 6NaCN \rightarrow \underset{\text{Sodium ferrocyanide}}{Na_4[Fe(CN)_6]} + 2NaOH$$

$$3Na_4[Fe(CN)_6] + 2Fe_2(SO_4)_3 \rightarrow Fe_4[Fe(CN)_6] + 6Na_2SO_4$$

Ferric ferrocyanide (Prussian blue colour)

(ii) For detection of sulphur

$$S + 2Na \rightarrow Na_2S$$

(a) Lead acetate test

$$Na_2S + (CH_3COO)_2Pb \rightarrow \underset{\text{Lead sulphide (black ppt.)}}{PbS\uparrow} + 2CH_3COONa$$

(b) Nitroprusside test

$Na_2S + Na_2\,[Fe(CN)_5NO] \rightarrow Na_4[Fe(CN)_5NOS]$

Sodium sulphonitro-prusside (violet)

(c) For detection of halogens

$X + Na \rightarrow NaX$, where X = Cl, Br, or I

$NaX + AgNO_3 \rightarrow AgX\downarrow + NaNO_3$

Q.10. Give the chemistry of silver mirror test of Tollen's reagent.

Ans. The organic compounds like aldehydes which are easily oxidisable give silver mirror test.

$R—CHO + 2Ag(NH_3)_2OH \rightarrow 2Ag\downarrow + R—COONH_4 + H_2O + 2NH_3$

Tollen's reagent (Silver mirror or grey ppt.)

or $R—CHO + Ag_2O \rightarrow 2Ag\downarrow + R—COOH$

Addition of aldehyde causes the reduction of silver ion to metallic silver which appears as a mirror on heating.

Q.11. Which aliphatic compounds burn with smoky flame and why?

Ans. Chloroform and carbon tetrachloride burn with a smoky flame, because these compounds on burning (oxidation) provide chlorine which reduces the approach of oxygen to oxidise the carbon to carbon monoxide and carbon dioxide. Hence, smoky flame is produced. Acetylene also burns with a smoky flame, because percentage of carbon in acetylene and benzene is same.

Q.12. What is chemically Baeyer's reagent?

Ans. 1% alkaline solution of $KMNO_4$ is termed as Baeyer's reagent.

Q.13. Why Baeyer's reagent is used in organic qualitative analysis?

Ans. Baeyer's reagent is used to detect the presence of unsaturation in the organic compounds.

Q.14. What is the function of bromine water in organic analysis?

Ans. Bromine water serves as a brominating agent or oxidising agent in organic analysis.

Q.15. What is the main difference between aqueous $FeCl_3$ and alcoholic $FeCl_3$ solution?

Ans. pH value is different in aqueous and alcoholic solutions of $FeCl_3$. Aqueous $FeCl_3$ solution undergoes hydrolysis and becomes acidic. Hence, it attains pH less than 7, while alcoholic $FeCl_3$ solution is almost neutral and has pH value equal to 7.

Q.16. Name the group which is common in aldehydes and ketones?

Ans. The carbonyl (C=O) group is common in aldehydes and ketones.

Q.17. Give the chemistry of Fehling's solution test for aldehyde.

Ans. Silver mirror test is given by the organic compounds like aldehydes, which are easily oxidisable. The following reaction occurs during the test :

$$R\text{—}CHO + \underset{\text{Tollen's reagent}}{2Ag(NH_3)_2OH} \rightarrow \underset{\text{(Silver mirror grey ppt.)}}{2Ag\downarrow} + R\text{—}COONH_4 + H_2O + 2NH_3$$

or

$$R\text{—}CHO + Ag_2O \rightarrow 2Ag\downarrow + R\text{—}COOH$$

Addition of aldehyde causes the reduction of silver ion to metallic silver which appears as a mirror on heating.

Q.18. Give the chemistry of $FeCl_3$ test with phenol (carbolic acid).

Ans. $$\underset{\text{Phenol}}{6C_6H_5OH} + FeCl_3 \rightarrow \underset{\text{(Violet coloured complex ion)}}{13H^+[Fe(OC_6H_5)_6]^{3-}} + 3HC1$$

Q.19. Give the chemistry of iodoform test for ketones.

Ans. $$R\text{—}COCH_3 + 3I_2 + 4NaOH \rightarrow \underset{\text{(Iodoform ppt.)}}{CHI_3} + R\text{—}COONa + 3H_2O + 3NaI$$

Q.20. Why dye test is performed at low temperature?

Ans. Diazonium chloride formed in the reaction during dye test is unstable and explosive at high temperature, therefore dye test is performed at low temperature.

Q.21. What is the effect of moisture and impurities on melting point or boiling point?

Ans. Presence of moisture and impurities lower the melting point while boiling point is elevated.

CHAPTER 2

Q.1. What is sodium bicarbonate test in carboxylic acids?

Ans. Carboxylic acids react with sodium bicarbonate. Vigorous evolution of CO_2 with brisk effervescence occurs confirming the presence of COOH group.

$$RCOOH + NaHCO_3 \rightarrow RCOONa + H_2O + CO_2\uparrow$$

Q.2. Write down ferric chloride test for phenolic group.

Ans. Phenols react with neutral ferric chloride solution and produce a violet, blue or green or wine red colour. The following reaction occurs :

$$6C_6H_5OH + FeCl_3 \rightarrow \underset{\text{Complex ion (violet)}}{3H^+[(C_6H_5O)_6Fe]^{3-}} + 3HCl$$

Q.3. Account for the following physical properties of carboxylic acids :

(a) Only carboxylic acids with 5 or fewer C's are soluble in water.

(b) Acetic acid in the vapour state shows a relative molecular mass of 120.

Ans. (a) RCOOH dissolves because H and COOH can form H-bond with water. The R portion is nonpolar and lyophobic: this effect predominates as R gets large (over 5 C's).

(b) CH_3COOH typically undergoes dimeric intermolecular H-bonding in the vapour state.

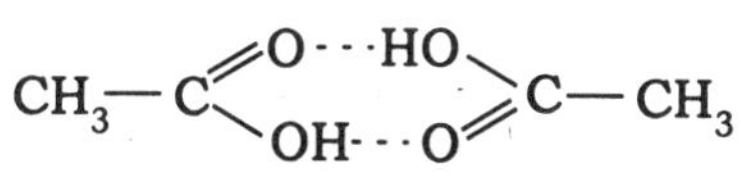

Q.4. Explain why highly branched carboxylic acids such as:

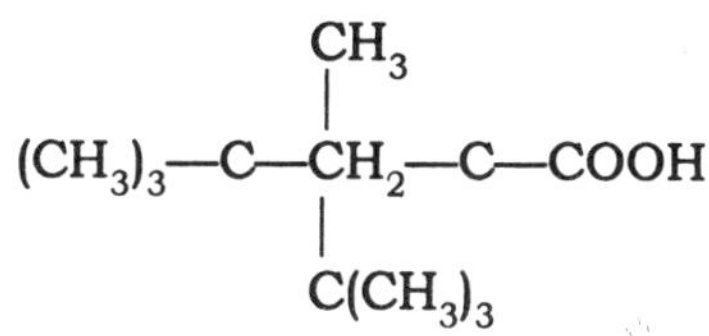

are less acidic than unbranched acids.

Ans. The $—CO_2^-$ group of the branched acid is shielded from the solvent molecules and cannot be stabilized by solvation as effectively as can acetate anion.

Q.5. Although p-hydroxybenzoic acid is less acidic than benzoic acid, salicylic (o-hydroxybenzoic) acid is 15 times more acidic than benzoic acid. Explain.

Ans. The enhanced acidity is partly due to very effective H-bonding in the conjugate base, which decreases its basic strength.

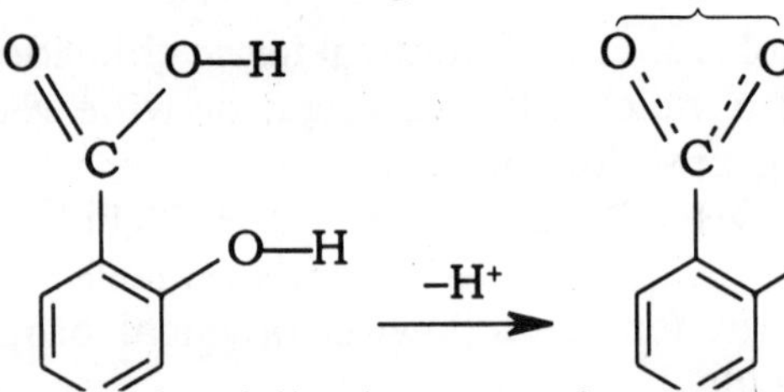

Q.6. Name the following organic compounds :

(a)

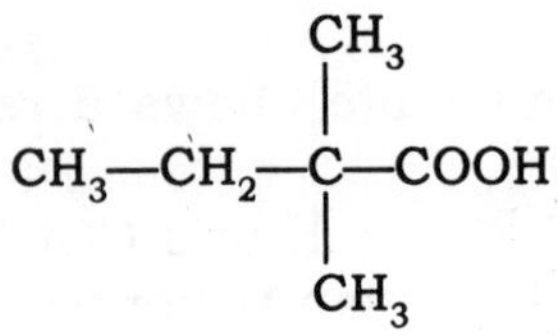

(b)

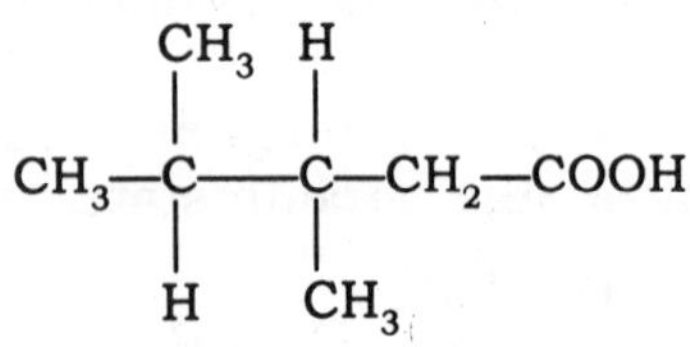

(c) $CH_3—CH = CH—CH = CH—COOH$

(d)

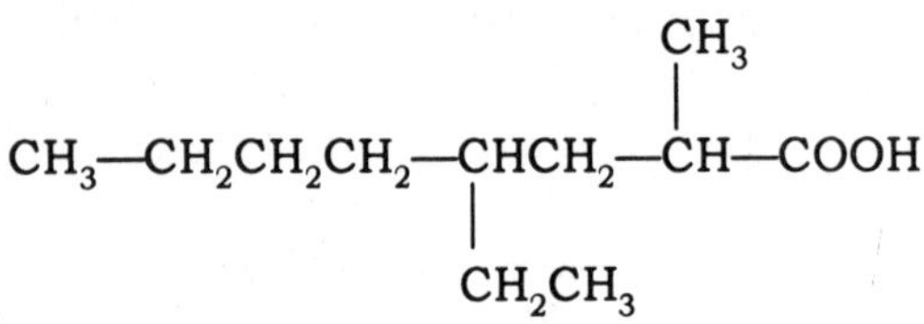

Ans. (a) Dimethylethylacetic acid or 2, 2-dimethylbutanoic acid.

(b) 3, 4-dimethylpentanoic acid or β, γ-dimethylvaleric acid.

(c) 2, 4-hexadienoic acid (sorbic acid).

(d) 4-ethyl-2-methyloctanoic acid.

Q.7. Distinguish by simple test tube reaction among hexane, hexanol and hexanoic acid.

Ans. (a) Only hexanoic acid liberates CO_2 from aqueous Na_2CO_3; (b) Na reacts with hexanol to liberate H_2; (c) while hexane is inert.

Q.8. Compare the products formed on heating the following dicarboxylic acids :

(a) Oxalic acid.

(b) Malonic acid.

(c) Succinic acid.

(d) Glutaric acid (1.5-pentane dioic acid).

(e) Longer chain HOOC—$(CH_2)_n$ COOH acids.

Ans. Acids (a) and (b) undergo decarboxylation while acids (c), (d) and (e) undergo dehydration.

(a) **Decarboxylation**

$$HOOC—COOH \xrightarrow{\text{Heat}} CO_2 + H—COOH \longrightarrow CO_2 + H_2O$$

(b) **Decarboxylation**

$$HOOC—CH_2—COOH \xrightarrow{\Delta} CO_2 + CH_3COOH$$

(c) Intramolecular dehydration and ring formation leading to formation of succinic anhydride.

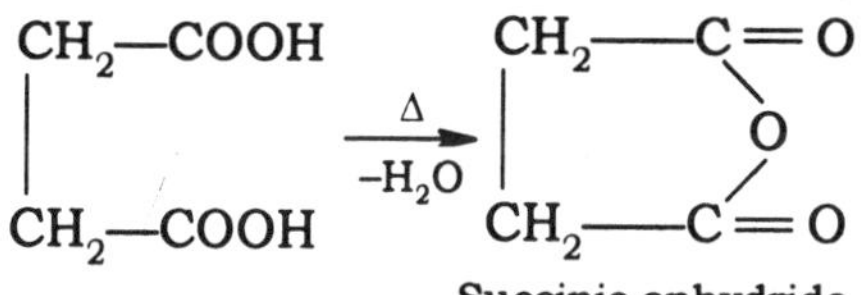

Succinic anhydride

(d) Intramolecular dehydration and ring formation leading to formation of glutaric anhydride.

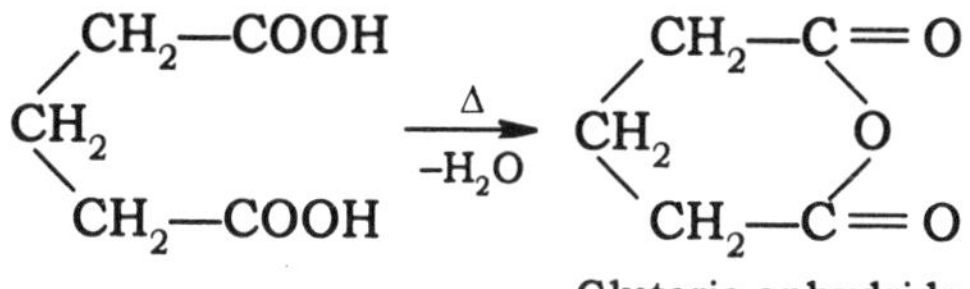

Glutaric anhydride

(e) Longer chain α, ω-dicarboxylic acids usually undergo intermolecular dehydration on heating to form long chain polymeric anhydrides. In the following equation, $n > 3$.

$$HOOC{-}(CH_2)_n{-}COOH \xrightarrow{\Delta} HOOC{-}(CH_2)_n{-}\underset{\displaystyle \overset{\|}{O}}{C}{-}O{-}\underset{\displaystyle \overset{\|}{O}}{C}{-}(CH_2)_n{-}\underset{\displaystyle \overset{\|}{O}}{C}{-}\ldots$$

Q.9. Name the following acid derivatives :

(a) C_6H_5COCl

(b) $CH_3CH_2{-}\underset{\displaystyle \overset{\|}{O}}{C}{-}NH_2$

(c) $CH_3CH_2{-}\underset{\displaystyle \overset{\|}{O}}{C}{-}O{-}\underset{\displaystyle \overset{\|}{O}}{C}{-}CH_2CH_3$

(d) $C_6H_5{-}\underset{\displaystyle \overset{\|}{O}}{C}{-}OC_6H_5$

(e) $CH_3CH_2CH_2{-}\underset{\displaystyle \overset{\|}{O}}{C}{-}OCH_2{-}CH_3$

(f) $C_6H_5CH_2COO{-}K^+$

Ans. (a) Benzoyl chloride.

(b) Propanamide or propionamide.

(c) Propionic or propanoic anhydride.

(d) Phenyl benzoate.

(e) Ethyl butyrate (butanoate).

(f) Potassium phenyl acetate.

Q.10. β-hydroxy acids undergo dehydration but do not yield a lactone. Give the structure of the product and account for its formation.

Ans.

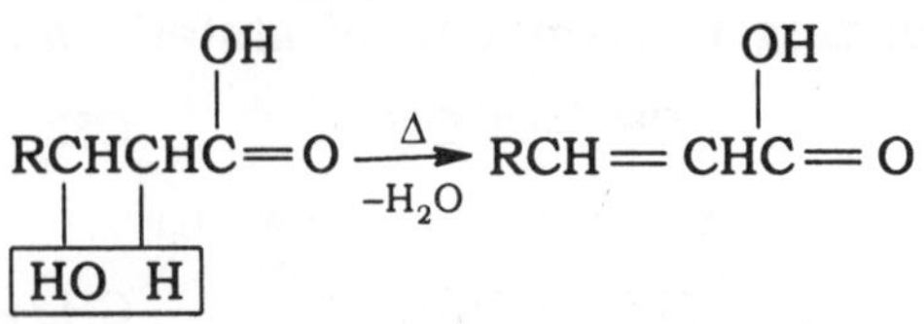

A double bond forms because the product is a stable, conjugated α, β-unsaturated acid.

Q.11. Distinguish by chemical tests the following :

(a) CH_3COCl from $(CH_3CO)_2O$

(b) Nitrobenzene from benzamide.

Ans. (a) With H_2O, CH_3COCI liberates HCl, which is detected by giving a white precipitate of AgCl on adding $AgNO_3$.

(b) Refluxing the amide with aqueous NaOH releases NH_3, which is detected by following tests :

(i) By odour.

(ii) With moist litmus.

(iii) By pH paper.

Q.12. What is nitroso reaction or Liebermann's test for phenolic group?

Ans. In a dry test tube take a little amount of phenolic compound and add few crystals of sodium nitrite $(NaNO_2)$. Heat the above mixture and cool it. Now add 1 ml of conc. H_2SO_4 and shake it. Deep green or blue colour is a positive test for phenolic group. Pour the mixture in excess of water, the colour will change to red to blue red. Add 20% sodium hydroxide (NaOH) solution. The colour of the mixture again turns deep green or blue. This reaction was suggested by Liebermann. The following reactions occur :

Step I : Phenol first reacts with nitrous acid that is formed from the nitrite to give p-nitrophenol :

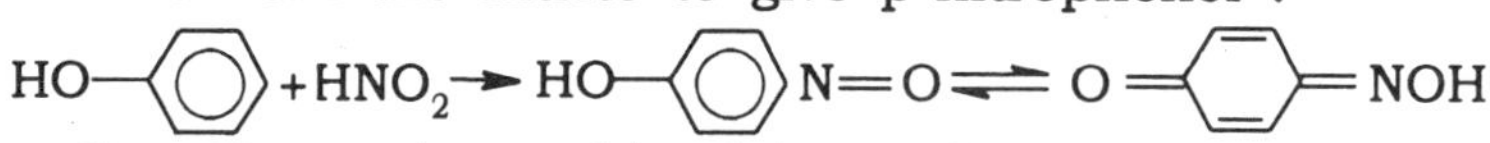

Step II : p-nitrosophenol is readily condensed with excess phenol to give phenolindophenol having the quinonoid structure :

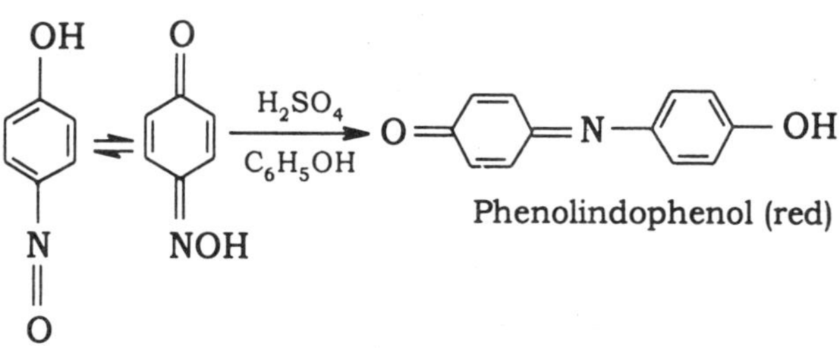

Phenolindophenol (red)

Blue

Step III : Phenol-indophenol reacts with acids and alkalis to give salts, in which the molecule of phenolindophenol turns into cation or anion respectively. These ions, whose structure is also quinonoid, colour the solution blue or green. When the acid solution is diluted with water, the solution is hydrolysed to liberate free red phenolindophenol.

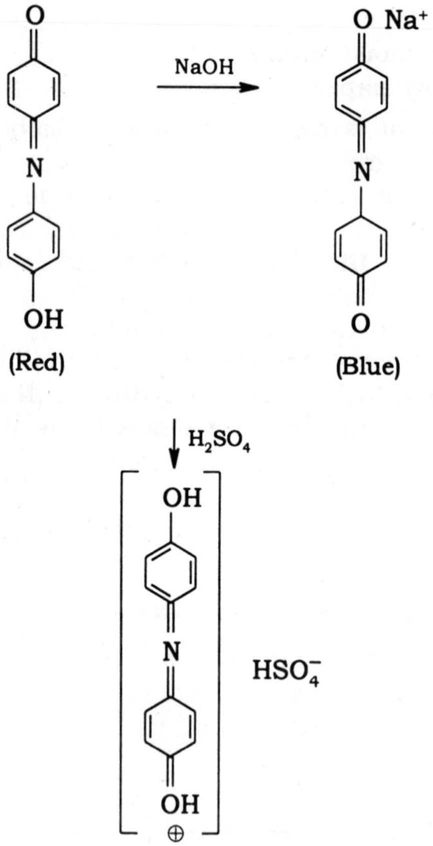

Q.13. Write structural formula for (a) phenol (b) p-cresol (c) resorcinol (d) catechol (e) hydroquinone (f) salicylic acid.

Ans.

(a)

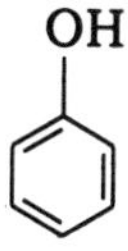

Phenol

(b)

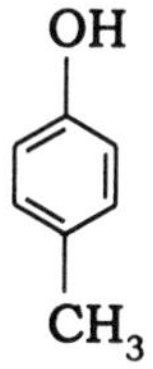

p-cresol

(c)

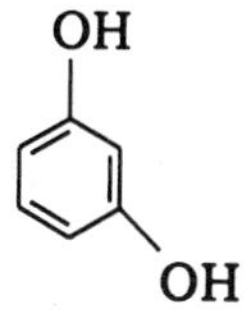

Resorcinol

(d)

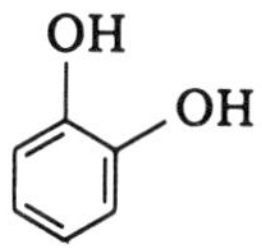

Catechol

(e)

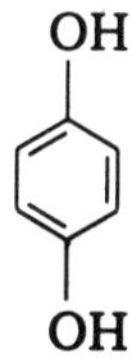

Hydroquinone

(f)

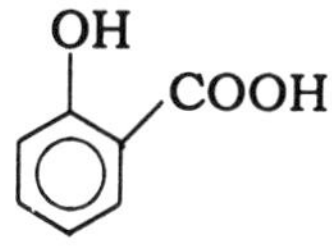

Salicylic acid

Q.14. Compared to toluene, phenol has higher boiling point and is more soluble in H_2O. Explain.

Ans. High boiling point and solubility of phenol in water can be explained on the basis of hydrogen bonding.

High boiling point is due to intermolecular H-bonding and solubility in water is due to H-bonding with H_2O.

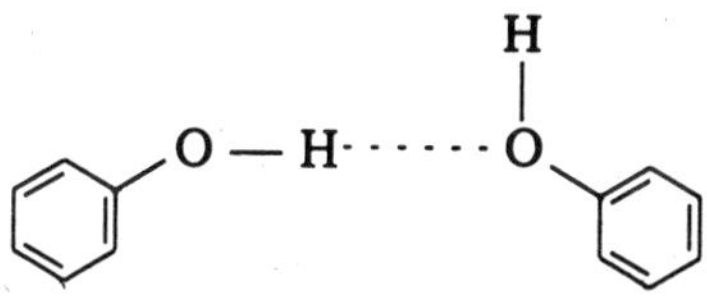

Intermolecular H-bonding

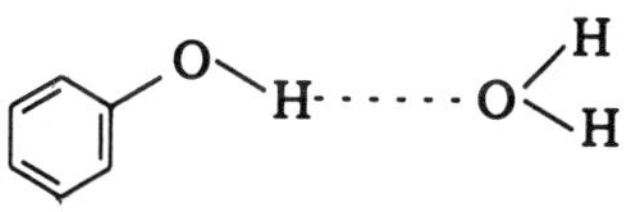

H-bonding with H_2O

Q.15. Why does aqueous $NaHCO_3$ solution dissolves RCOOH but not C_6H_5OH?

Ans. In both cases the product would be carbonic acid, which is a stronger acid than phenols, but weaker than carboxylic acids. Acid-base equilibria lie towards the weaker acid and weaker base.

Q.16. How neutral ferric chloride ($FeCl_3$) solution is prepared.

Ans. Add dil ammonium hydroxide solution (NH_4OH) drop by drop in $FeCl_3$ solution until precipitates are formed. Filter it. Use the filtrate for the test.

Q.17. Write down the reaction of alcohol with sodium metal.

Ans. $2R\text{—}OH + 2Na \longrightarrow 2R\text{—}ONa + H_2\uparrow$ Alcohol

Q.18. Write down the reaction of alcohol with ceric ammonium nitrate solution.

Ans.

$$\underset{\text{Alcohol}}{2R\text{—}OH} + \underset{\text{Ceric ammonium nitrate}}{(NH_4)_2[Ce(NO_3)_6]} \longrightarrow \underset{\text{Red colouration}}{[Ce(NO_3)_4(ROH)_2]} + 2NH_4NO_3$$

Q.19. What is 2, 4-DNP?

Ans. It is 2, 4-dinitrophenyl hydrazine.

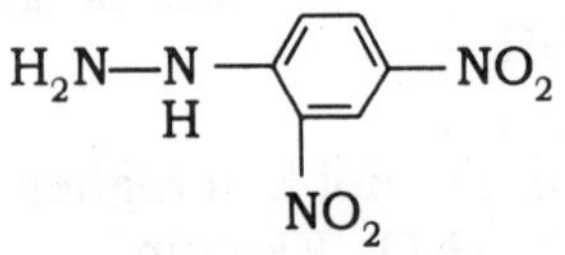

2,4-dinitrophenyl hydrazine

Q. 20. What is Tollen's reagent?

Ans. Tollen's reagent is ammoniacal silver nitrate solution. It is prepared by adding dil. NaOH solution to 1 ml of $AgNO_3$ solution. The white precipitate, thus produced is dissolved by adding a few drops of ammonium hydroxide. This reagent should be prepared fresh when needed.

$$AgNO_3 + NaOH \longrightarrow \underset{\text{Soluble in ammonia}}{AgOH\downarrow} + NaNO_3$$

Q.21. What is Schiffs reagent and where is it used?

Ans. Schiffs reagent is also known as fuchsin-aldehyde reagent. It is prepared by passing sulphur dioxide gas in 1% solution of fuchsin (rosaniline hydrochloride) till its colour is discharged.

Fuchsin (rosaniline) is a derivative of triphenylmethane.

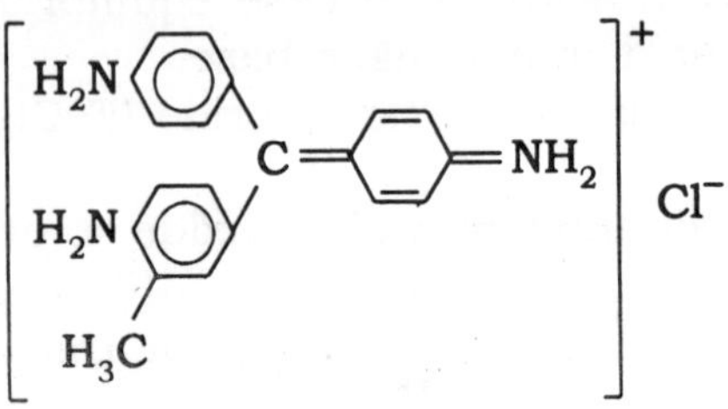

(Rosaniline hydrochloride)

Its red colour is due to the quinonoid structure. As two molecules of sulphurous acid are joined to fuchsin, a colourless compound is formed. The quinonoid grouping is absent from Schiffs reagent.

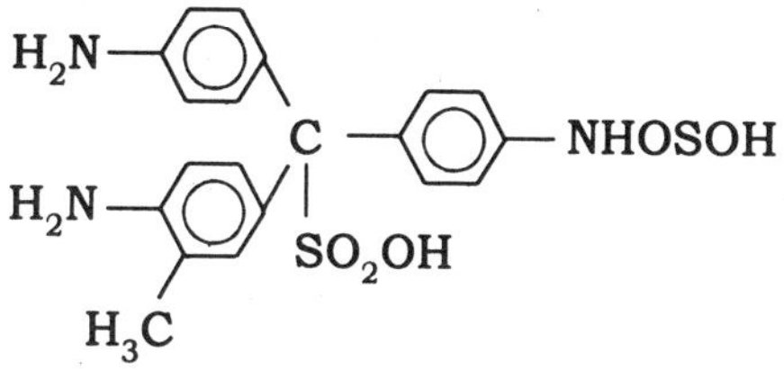

Schiff's reagent

Schiffs reagent is used to detect aldehyde group. As aldehydes combine with Schiffs reagent, the structure is altered and new substances are formed, whose structure is quinonoid. Their colour is therefore the same as that of fuchsin, except that the new is deeper blue.

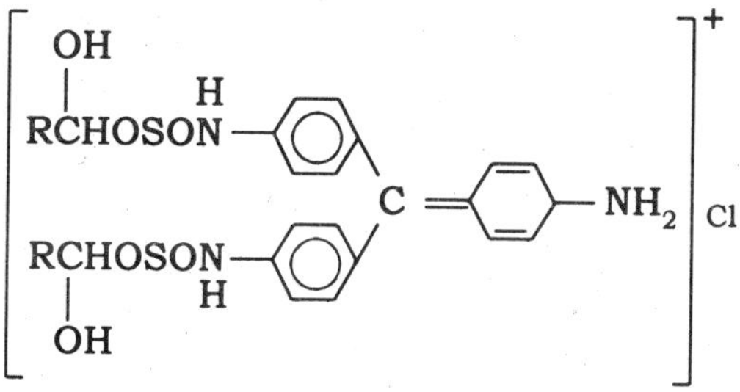

These compounds react gradually with excess sulphurous anhydride to eliminate aldehyde as its bisulphite compound and convert back to free Schiffs reagent. The solution is therefore decolourised on standing.

Q.22. What is Fehling's solution and where is it used?

Ans. Fehling's solution is a mixture of copper sulphate and sodium hydroxide along with the solution of sodium potassium tartrate (Seignette salt).

Fehling's solution A : Copper sulphate (3.5 g of $CuSO_4$ $5H_2O$ in 50 ml of water).

Fehling's solution B : Sodium potassium tartrate in water alkali solution (17.3 g of Seignette's salt and 6 g of sodium hydroxide in 50 ml water).

A molecule of tartrate contains two adjacent hydroxyl groups containing mobile hydrogen atoms. The tartrate therefore reacts with copper hydroxide in an alkaline medium to give soluble copper complexes. These complexes containing divalent copper easily oxidize many aldehydes and sugars to precipitate cuprous oxide and partly metallic copper. Fehling's solution contains K^+, Na^+ ion and the complex anion in an alkaline medium.

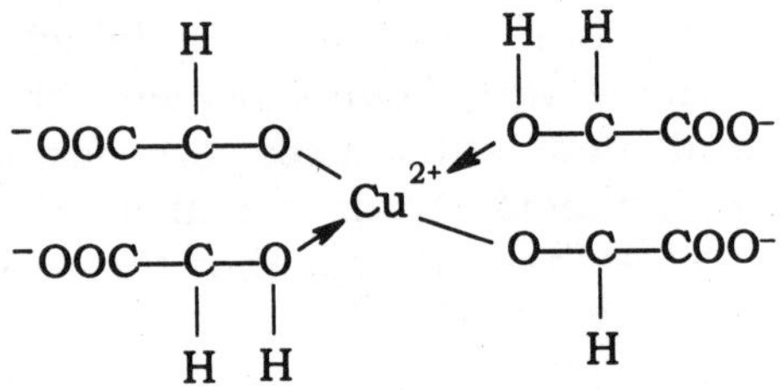

Monovalent copper does not form this complex with tartrate.

Q.23. Write down the chemistry of iodoform test given by ketones containing $-\overset{O}{\overset{\|}{C}}-CH_3$ group.

Ans. $NaOCl + H_2O + 2KI \rightarrow NaOH + KOH + I_2 + KCl$

Sodium hypochloride

$CH_3COCH_3 + 3I_2 + NaOH \rightarrow CHI_3 + CH_3COONa + 3NaI + 3H_2O$

Acetone — Iodoform (yellow crystals)

Q.24. Why formaldehyde does not give iodoform test?

Ans. Formaldehyde molecule does not contain the atom grouping $\left(-\overset{\|}{C}-CH_3\right)$ that is necessary for the formation of iodoform. For this reason formaldehyde is oxidized to formic acid in the conditions of the experiment.

Q.25. Why ethyl aceto-acetate does not give iodoform test although it contains $-\overset{\overset{\Large O}{\|}}{C}-CH_3$ group?

Ans. Under the conditions of the experiment, ethyl aceto-acetate decomposed with liberation of acetic acid, the methyl group of which is not easily iodized.

Q.26. Write down the reaction of carbonyl group with 2, 4-dinitrophenyl hydrazine (2,4-DNP).

Ans.

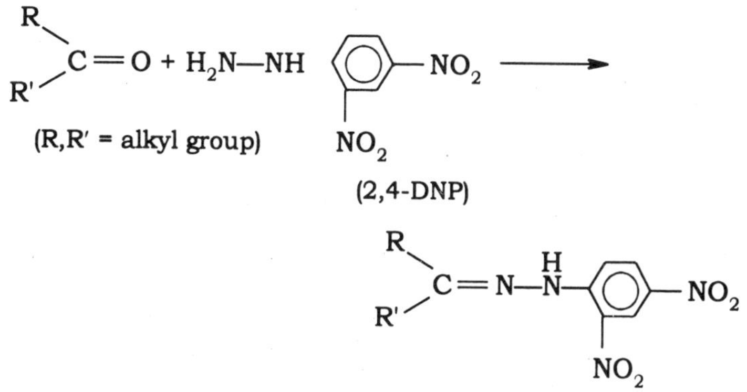

(2,4-dinitrophenyl hydrazone)

Q.27. Give the chemistry of hydroxamic acid test for ester group (—COOR).

Ans. Esters on treatment with hydroxylamine are converted into hydroxamic acids.

$$\underset{\text{Ester}}{RCOOR'} + \underset{\text{Hydroxylamine}}{NH_2OH} \rightarrow \underset{\text{Hydroxamic acid}}{RCONHOH} + R'\text{–}OH$$

Hydroxamic acid on treatment with ferric ions produce deep red or red violet coloured ferric hydroxamates.

$$3RCONHOH + FeCl_3 \rightarrow \underset{\substack{\text{Ferric hydroxamate}\\ \text{(red violet)}}}{(RCONHO)_3Fe} + 3HCl$$

Q.28. Write down the chemistry of Mulliken's test for nitro group.

Ans. Nitro group in the presence of calcium chloride and zinc dust reduced to –NHOH (hydroxyl amine).

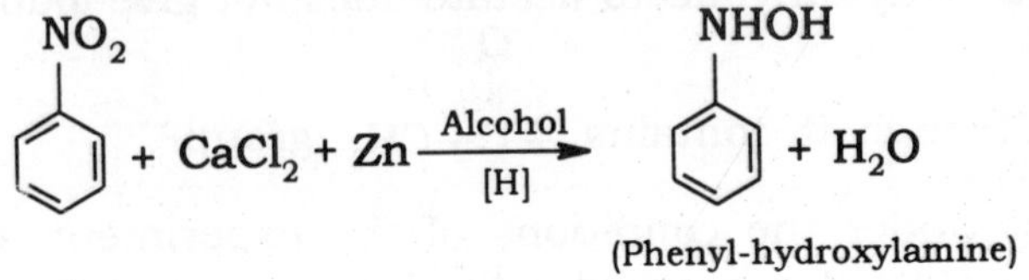

Hydroxyl amine group reduces Tollen's reagent.

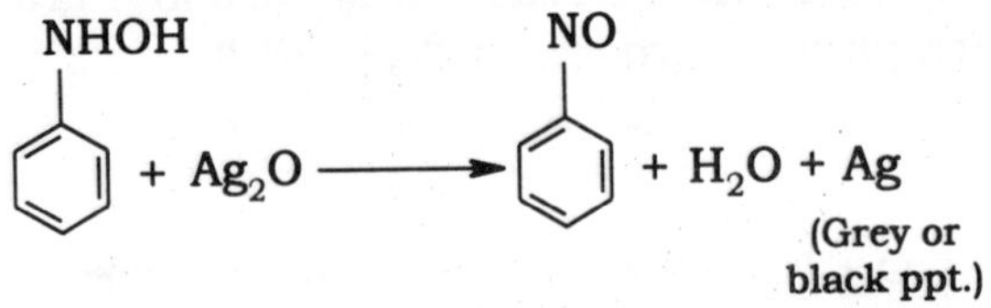

Q.29. What is carbylamine test or isocyanide test?

Ans. In this test primary amine reacts with chloroform in the presence of alcoholic sodium or potassium hydroxide. Warm it. A very bad smell of carbylamine (isocyanide) is obtained.

$$R\text{–}NH_2 + CHCl_3 + 3KOH \rightarrow \underset{\text{Isocyanide}}{R\text{–}NC} + 3KCl + 3H_2O$$

[After performing this test, destroy the mixture or isocyanide by adding excess of conc. HCl; the isocyanide would be hydrolysed to the odourless amine and throw it out.]

Q.30. Distinguish between aliphatic and aromatic primary amines.

Ans. Aromatic primary amines give diazonium salts with nitrous acid, which can be detected by formation of red dye with alkaline phenol solution.

Q.31. Give the chemistry of dye test for aromatic primary amines.

Ans. Aromatic primary amine reacts with nitrous acid (which is generated from $NaNO_2$ and HCl) and form diazonium salt at low temperature 0-5°C. Diazonium chloride forms red dye with alkaline β-naphthol solution at low temperature.

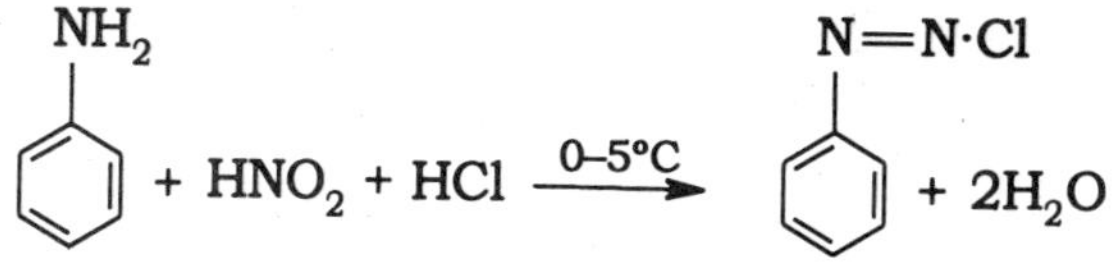

(Aniline) ($NaNO_2$ + HCl) (Diazonium chloride)

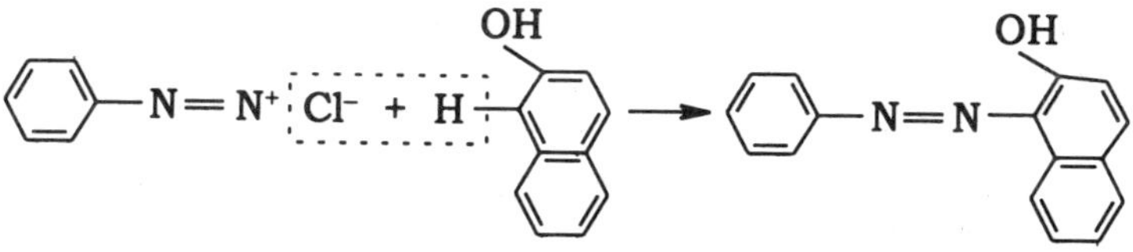

(β-naphthol) (Azo dye) (orange-red dye)

Q.32. What is osazone?

Ans. Carbohydrates which have a functional carbonyl group give osazone with phenyl hydrazine. This serves as a suitable derivative for characterization of carbohydrates.

$$\begin{array}{l} CHO \\ | \\ CHOH \\ | \\ R \end{array} \xrightarrow{H_2N\cdot NHPh} \begin{array}{l} CH{=}N\cdot NHPh \\ | \\ CHOH \\ | \\ R \end{array} \xrightarrow{PhNHNH_2} \begin{array}{l} CH{=}N\cdot NHPh \\ | \\ CO \\ | \\ R \end{array} + Ph\cdot NH_2 + NH_3$$

$$\begin{array}{l} CH{=}NNHPh \\ | \\ CHOH \\ | \\ R \end{array} \xrightarrow{Ph\cdot NHNH_2} \begin{array}{l} CH{=}N\cdot NHPh \\ | \\ CH{=}N\cdot NHPh \\ | \\ R \end{array}$$

Osazone

CHAPTERS 3 AND 4

Q.1. What is melting point?

Ans. The melting point of a compound is constant temperature, at which the solid and liquid phase are in equilibrium at one atmospheric pressure.

Q.2. The melting point is a very important characteristic (constant) of a solid substance. Why?

Ans. Because it can be used to identify an organic substance. It is the characteristic of substance purity. If a substance melts at a temperature below or higher than its true melting point, this indicates the presence of impurities.

Q.3. Why carbohydrates and amino acids do not have a fixed melting point?

Ans. Because these substances melt with decomposition within a wider range of temperatures. Some substances are charred or volatilized without melting.

Q.4. Why conc. H_2SO_4 is used as a bath for determining the melting point?

Ans. Because it has a high boiling point. If the working liquid is conc. sulphuric acid, the apparatus can be heated to 240-250°C, and re-used many times. When the acid darkens, add a pinch of KNO_3 (only two or three crystals) to decolourise it. A bath of conc. H_2SO_4 can be used for 3-4 months; during this time it can absorb much water from the air and its boiling point can decrease to 200°C and below.

Q.5. What is boiling point?

Ans. The boiling point of a liquid is that temperature at which the vapour pressure of a liquid is equal to the atmospheric pressure; the liquid boils freely at this temperature.

Q.6. Why boiling point is important?

Ans. The boiling point is an important constant of a substance. The boiling point, and also the range of temperature within which the substance is distilled, characterize the purity of a substance and can be used for its identification.

CHAPTER 5

Q.1. Write down the structures of (a) sulphanilamide, (b) sulphadiazine, (c) sulphacetamide, and (d) phthalylsulphathiazole.

Ans.

(a) 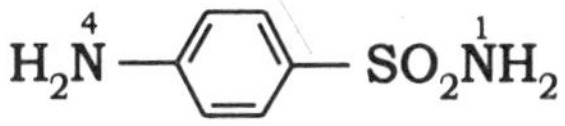

Sulphanilamide

Substitutions made in the amide NH_2 group (the N of which has been designated as N) have variable effects on anti-bacterial activity of the molecule. The para-NH_2 group (the N of which has been designated as N) is essential and can be replaced only by such radicals as can be converted in the tissues to a free amino group.

(b) 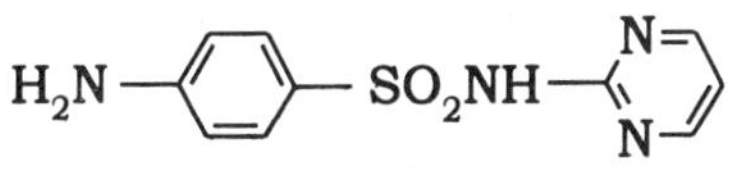

(Sulphadiazine)

(c) 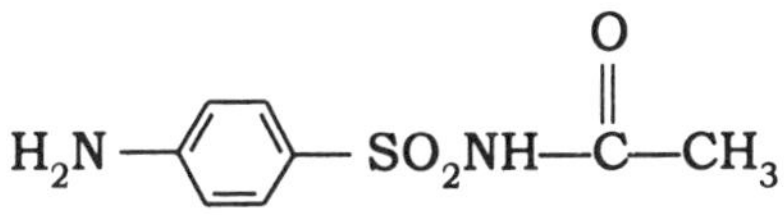

(Sulphacetamide)

(d) 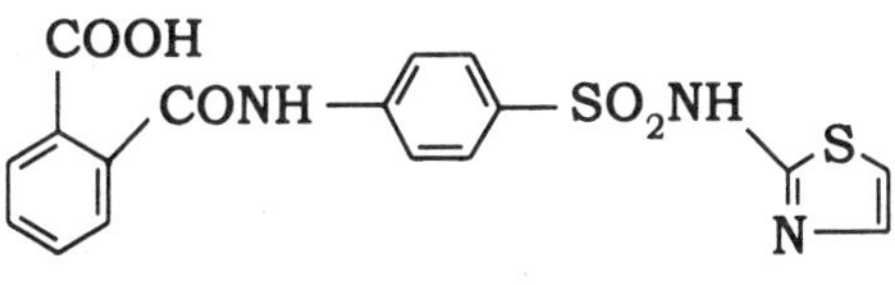

(Phthalylsulphathiazole)

Q.2. What happens when sulphadiazine is treated with alkaline copper sulphate solution?

Ans. When sulphadiazine is treated with alkaline copper sulphate solution, an olive green precipitate is formed, which becomes purple grey on standing. This is due to the fact that many of the sulphanilamides form coloured complexes with copper.

Q.3. What happens when aqueous solution of sulphacetamide sodium is treated with acetic acid?

Ans. When aqueous solution of sulphacetamide sodium is treated with acetic acid, it gives a white precipitate of free sulphacetamide and its melting point is determined for identification (Literature value 182-184°C).

Q.4. Write down the chemical reaction when sulphacetamide is heated with alcohol and sulphuric acid?

Ans.

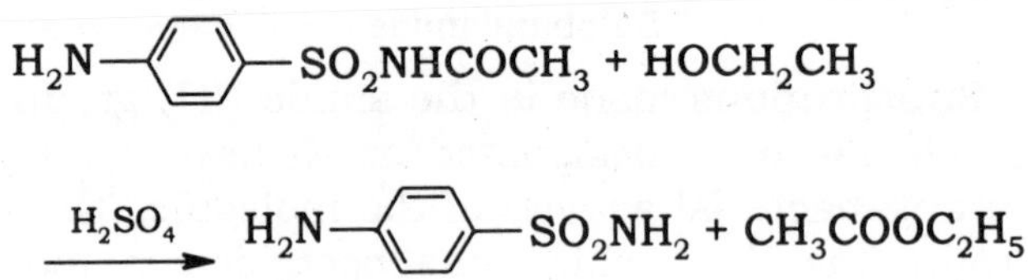

(Sulphanilamide) (Ethyl acetate)

Q.5. Write down the azo dye formation test with sulphanilamide?

Ans. The sulphanilamide having free p-NH_2 group (N^4) are primary aromatic amines. They can be diazotized into diazonium salts. The diazonium salts so formed are coupled with β-naphthol solution to give azo dye.

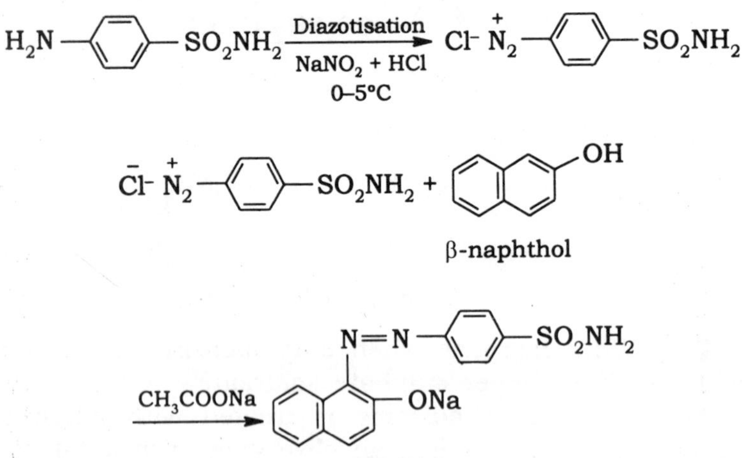

(An azo dye)

Q.6. Write down the azo dye formation test with sulphacetamide?

Ans.

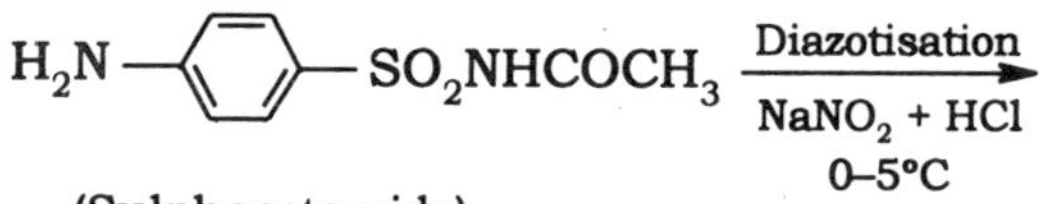

(Sulphacetamide)

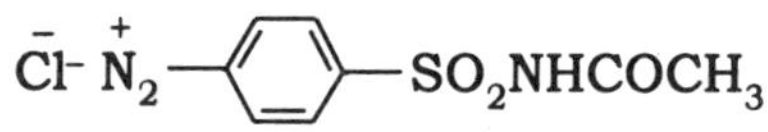

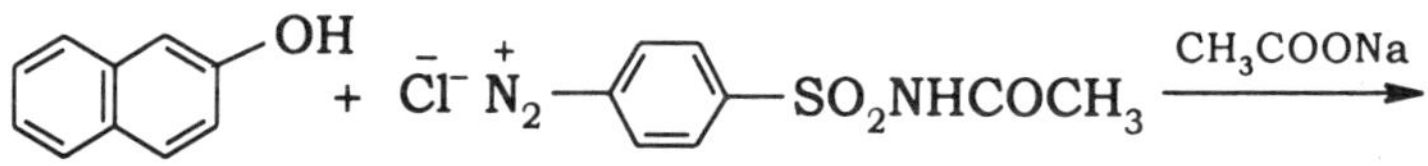

(β-naphthol)

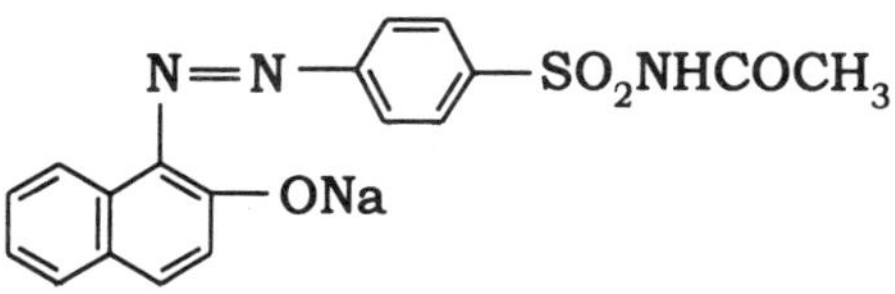

(An azo dye)

Q.7. What happens when phthalylsulphathiazole is heated strongly in a dry test tube? If moistened lead acetate paper is placed on the mouth of the test tube what colour change you will observe?

Ans. Phthalylsulphathiazole decomposes on strong heating and gives pungent vapours. The vapours blacken moistened lead acetate paper due to the presence of hydrogen sulphide.

$$H_2S + Pb(OOCCH_3)_2 \rightarrow PbS\downarrow + 2CH_3COOH$$

(Black ppt.)

Q.8. Write structures of products formed on alkaline hydrolysis of phthalylsulphathiazole?

Ans. Phthalylsulphathiazole on alkaline hydrolysis gives sulphathiazole and phthalic acid.

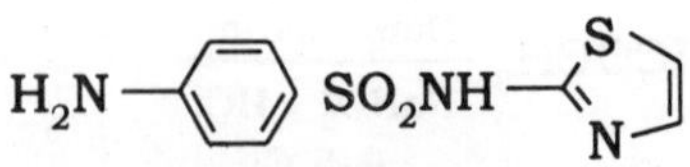

(Sulphathiazole)

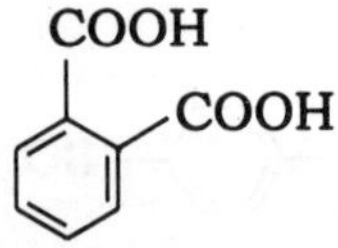

(Phthalic acid)

Q.9. What happens when phthalylsulphathiazole is heated with resorcinol and sulphuric acid?

Ans. Phthalylsulphathiazole on heating with resorcinol and sulphuric acid forms fluorescein dye, which in alkaline solution (10% NaOH solution) gives a distinct green fluorescence. The fluorescence disappears when the solution is made acidic, but reappears when it is made alkaline.

Q.10. Write down the structure of barbituric acid.

Ans.

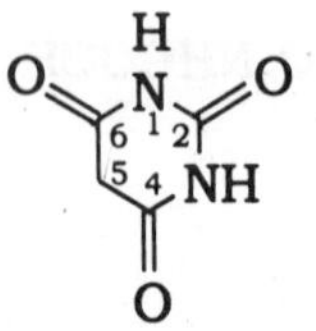

Barbituric acid
(2,4,6-trioxohexahydropyrimidine)

Q.11. Write down the structure of (a) amylobarbitone, and (b) amylobarbitone sodium.

Ans. (a)

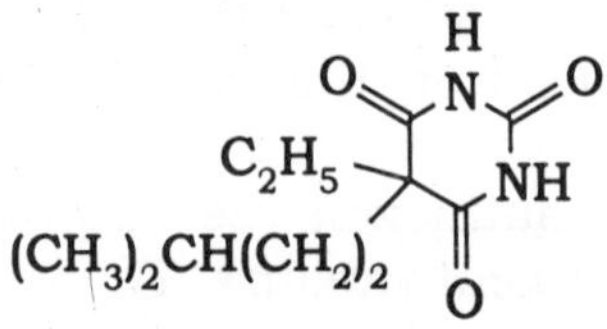

Amylobarbitone or
5-ethyl-5-isopentylbarbituric acid

(b)

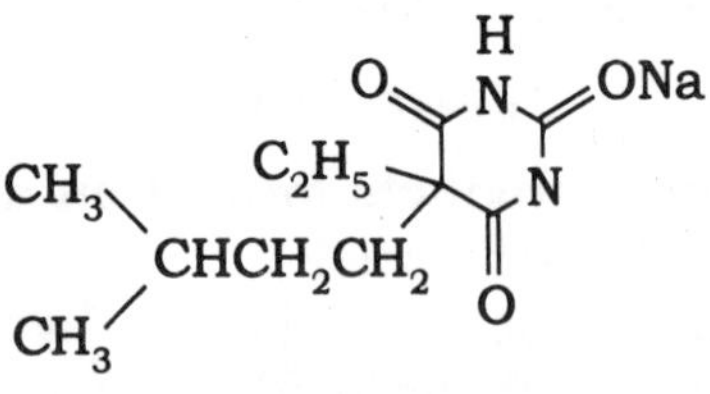

Amylobarbitone sodium or sodium salt
of 5-ethyl-5-isopentylbarbituric acid

Q.12. How will you synthesize barbituric acid?

Ans. Barbituric acid is the condensation product of urea and malonic acid.

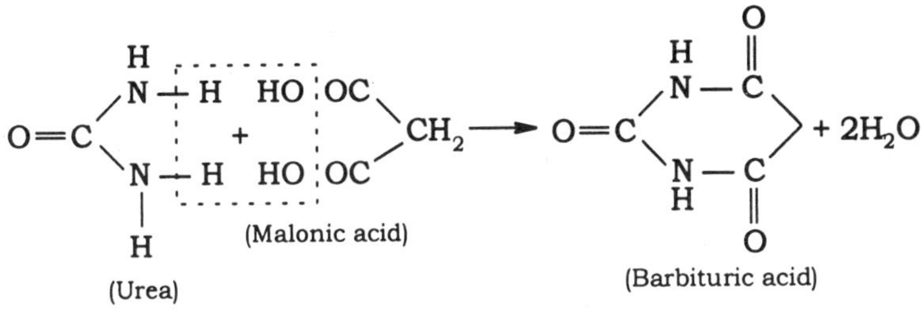

Q.13. Explain the acidic character of barbituric acid.

Ans. Barbituric acid has acidic character, because the keto form (—CO—NH) is in equilibrium with the enol form (—C[OH] : N—) the hydrogen of which readily dissociates.

Q. 14. Write down the structural formula of (a) phenothiazines, and (b) chlorpromazine hydrochloride.

Ans. (a)

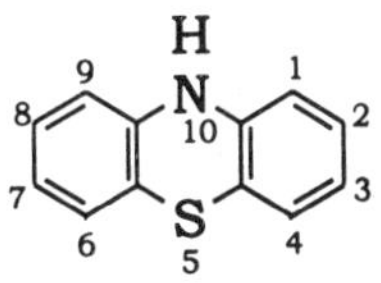

(Phenothiazine)

(b)

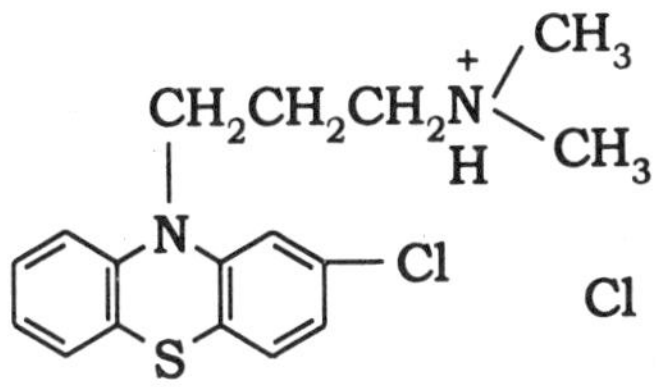

(Chlorpromazine hydrochloride)

CHAPTER 6

Q.1. What is acetylation ?

Ans. The replacement of an active hydrogen by an acetyl group is known as acetylation, e.g. the replacement of active hydrogen of compounds containing —OH (alcohols and phenols), —NH_2 (primary amines) and —NH (secondary amines) group.

$$\underset{\text{Phenol}}{C_6H_5O}\,\boxed{H + Cl}\,\underset{\text{Acetyl chloride}}{COCH_3} \xrightarrow{\text{Pyridine}} \underset{\text{Phenyl acetate}}{C_6H_5O\cdot CO\ CH_3} + HCl$$

Pyridine absorbs the hydrogen chloride formed during the reaction.

Q.2. What are the important uses of acetylation?

Ans. Acetylation is useful in:

(i) The protection of —OH or —NH_2 groups in many reactions, it is desirable to protect these groups from the reaction intended for the other groups in the molecule. So firstly convert these —OH or —NH_2 group into its acetyl derivative perform the required reactions. The free —OH or —NH_2 group can be regenerated by the hydrolysis at the end of the reaction.

(ii) The preparation of mono-substituted derivatives. For example, bromination of aniline or phenol gives tribromoaniline or tribromophenol respectively. If, however, the amino group of aniline is protected by acetylation, the resulting compound mainly form p-bromoacetanilide. The later on hydrolysis gives p-bromoaniline.

Q.3. What is benzoylation?

Ans. The introduction of a benzoyl group (C_6H_5CO—) in place of the active hydrogen of —OH, —NH_2 or >NH group is known as benzoylation, e.g.

$$\underset{\text{Aniline}}{C_6H_5NH_2} + \underset{\text{Benzoyl chloride}}{C_6H_5COCl} \xrightarrow{\text{NaOH}} \underset{\text{Benzanilide}}{C_6H_5NH\cdot CO\cdot C_6H_5} + HCl$$

Q.4. What are the advantages of benzoylation over acetylation?

Ans. Benzoyl derivatives are crystalline solids with higher melting points than corresponding acetyl derivatives. Moreover, benzoyl derivatives can be easily prepared in aqueous solvents as unlike acetyl chloride or acetic anhydride, benzoyl chloride is very slowly hydrolysed by water.

Q.5. What is bromination?

Ans. Aromatic hydrocarbons and their substituted derivatives on treatment with bromine form appropriate bromo-substituted derivatives, e.g.

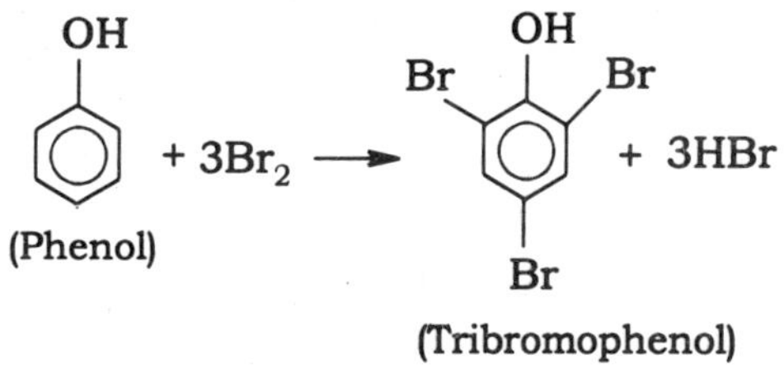

Q.6. What is diazotization?

Ans. Aromatic primary amines, having $-NH_2$ group directly attached to the nucleus, on treatment with nitrous acid in cold (0-5°C) yield diazonium salts. The reaction is known as diazotization.

$$C_6H_5NH_2 + NaNO_2 + 2HCl \xrightarrow{0\text{-}5°C} C_6H_5N_2^+Cl^- + NaCl + H_2O$$

Benzene diazonium chloride

Q.7. What is meant by nitration?

Ans. Aromatic hydrocarbon or their substituted derivatives, when treated with the mixture of conc. nitric acid and conc. sulphuric acid undergo nitration. In the nitration process, hydrogen atom or atoms are replaced by $—NO_2$ group or groups. In some cases nitration can be carried out even in the absence of sulphuric acid.

$$H_2SO_4 + HNO_3 \longrightarrow \overset{+}{N}O_2 + H_3O^+ + 2HSO_4$$

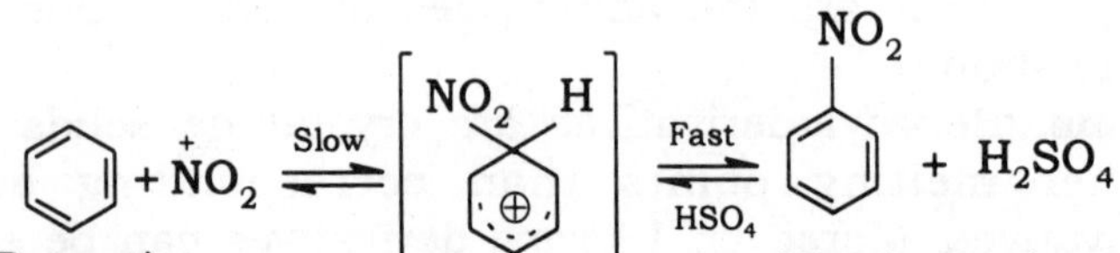

(Benzene) (Nitro benzene)

σ-complex
or
(Cyclopentadienyl
cation)

Q.8. Write down the chemical reaction for the preparation of aspirin from salicylic acid. What is the chemical name of aspirin?

Ans.

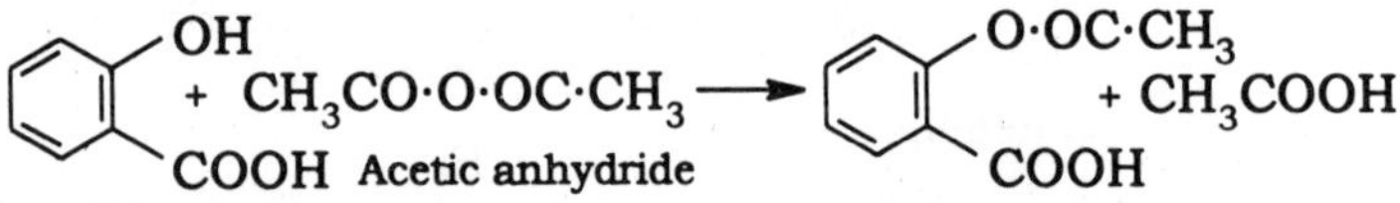

(Salicylic acid) Aspirin or acetylsalicylic acid

Chemical name is acetyl salicylic acid.

Q.9. What products would you get on hydrolyzing aspirin? Write down the chemical reaction.

Ans. When aspirin is boiled with NaOH and then acidified with HCl, salicylic acid is obtained.

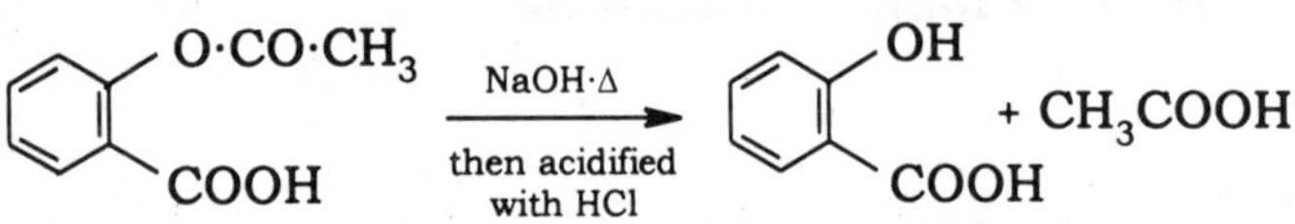

(Aspirin) (Salicylic acid)

Q.10. What is hippuric acid?

Ans. Hippuric acid is benzoyl glycine.

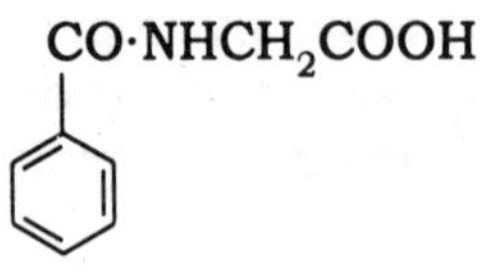

(Hippuric acid)

Q.11. What is picric acid?

Ans. Picric acid is 2, 4, 6-trinitrophenol.

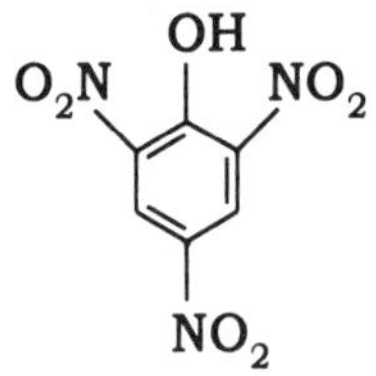

Q.12. Write down the structure of methyl orange.

Ans.

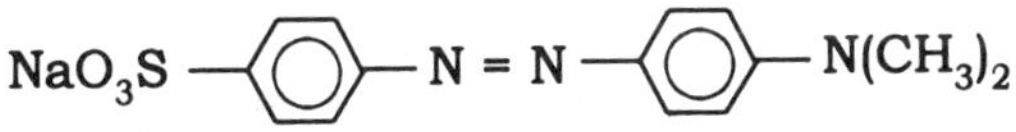

Methyl orange

Q.13. Write down the structure of phenolphthalein.

Ans.

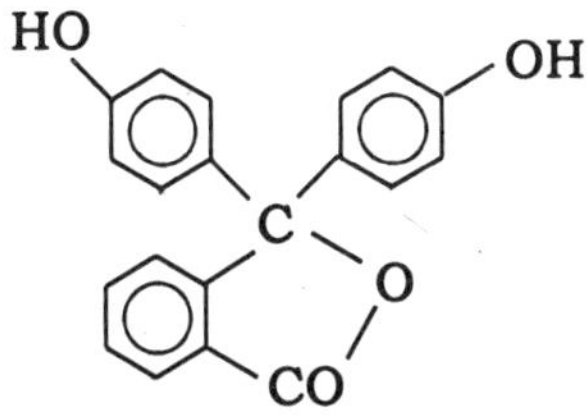

Phenolphthalein

Q.14. Write down the chemical reactions involved in the preparation of p-bromoacetanilide from aniline.

Ans. *Step I.*

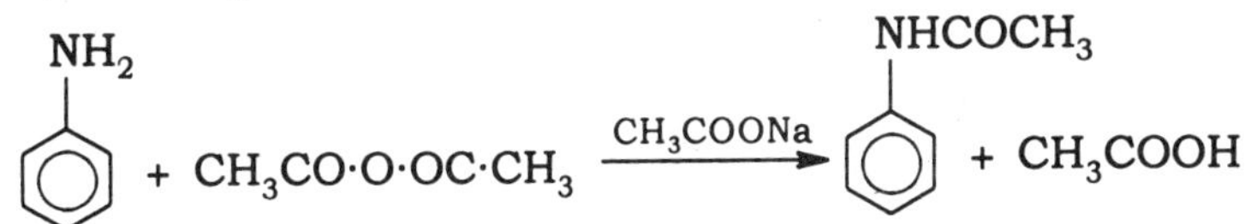

(Aniline) (Acetanilide)

Step II.

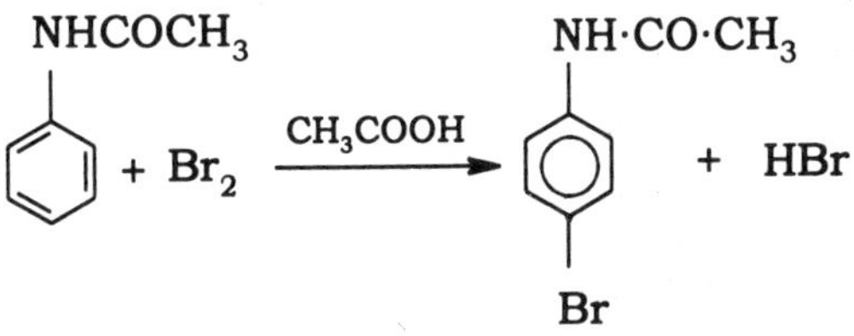

Q.15. Write Schotten-Baumann reaction for the preparation of benzanilide from aniline.

Ans. Aniline reacts with benzoyl chloride and gives benzanilide, the reaction is known as Schotten-Baumann reaction.

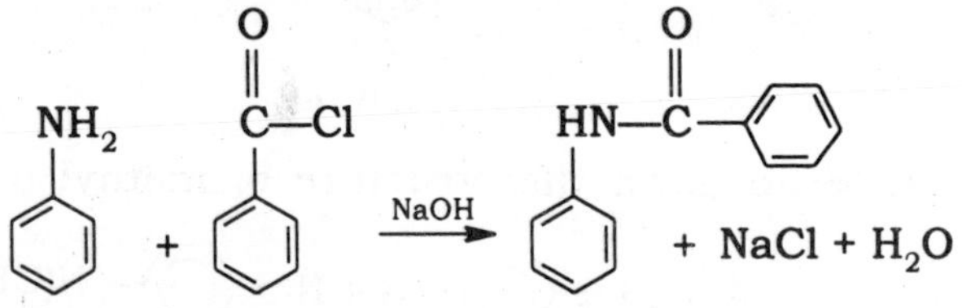

(Aniline) (Benzoyl chloride) (Benzanilide)

Q.16. What do you mean by oxidation and reduction reaction in organic chemistry?

Ans. A reaction which proceeds by the addition of oxygen is called *oxidation*. A reaction which proceeds by the addition of hydrogen is called reduction.

Q.17. Write down the reaction involved in the oxidation of benzoin by nitric acid.

Ans. Benzoin is oxidised by conc. HNO_3 to form benzil.

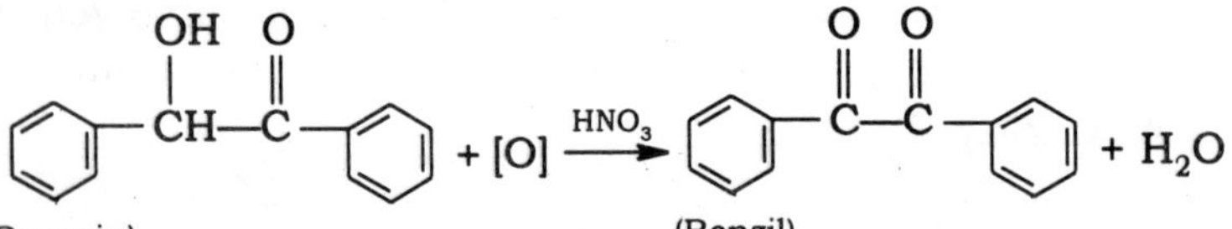

(Benzoin) (Benzil)

Q.18. What will be the product when anthracene is subjected to oxidation by a mixture of sodium dichromate and conc. H_2SO_4.

Ans. Anthracene gives 9,10-anthraquinone on oxidation by sodium dichromate and conc. H_2SO_4.

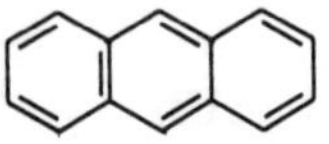

$+ Na_2Cr_2O_7 + 4H_2SO_4 \longrightarrow$

(Anthracene) (Sodium dichromate)

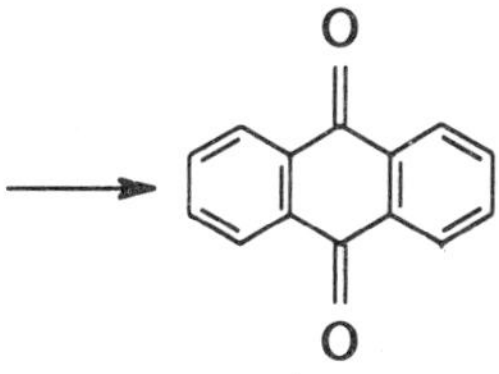 $+ Na_2SO_4 + Cr_2(SO_4)_3 + 5H_2O$

(9,10-anthraquinone)

Q.19. Write down the product formed when benzophenone is reduced by zinc dust and alcoholic NaOH.

Ans. Reduction of benzophenone with a zinc dust and alcoholic NaOH, a mild reducing agent gives benzhydrol (a secondary alcohol)

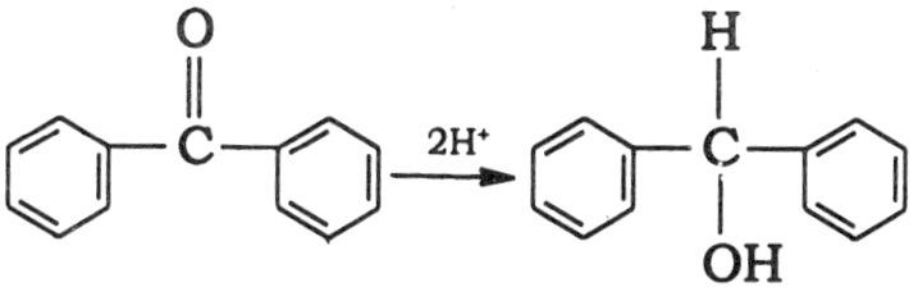

(Benzophenone) (Benzhydrol)

Q.20. Why is oxime formation important in organic chemistry?

Ans. Oxime formation is important because:

(i) They have sharp melting point so they are used to characterise the parent aldehydes and ketones.

(ii) Impure aldehydes and ketones can be purified by conversion into oximes and then recrystallisation and hydrolysis of oxime gives pure aldehydes and ketones.

(iii) Reduction of oxime gives pure primary amines.

Q.21. What is esterification?

Ans. When a monocarboxylic acid is heated with an alcohol in the presence of a small amount of mineral acid (H_2SO_4), it yields an ester and water, e.g.

$$\underset{\text{(Acetic acid)}}{CH_3COOH} + \underset{\text{(Ethanol)}}{HOC_2H_5} \underset{}{\overset{H^+}{\rightleftharpoons}} \underset{\text{(Ethylacetate)}}{CH_3COOC_2H_5} + H_2O$$

This reaction is known as *esterification.*

Q.22. What will be the hydrolysis product of p-bromoacetanilide by KOH and H_2O?

Ans. p-bromoacetanilide on hydrolysis by KOH and H_2O gives p-bromoaniline.

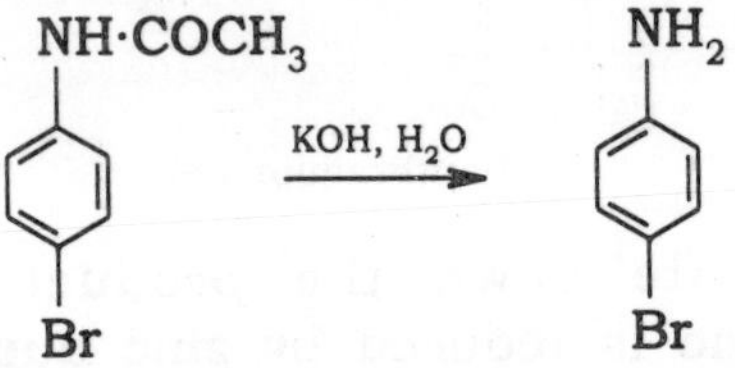

(p-bromoacetanilide) (p-bromoaniline)

Q.23. What is diazotisation?

Ans. Aromatic amines when treated with nitrous acid in cold mineral acid solution, yield aryldiazonium salts, e.g. aniline reacts with nitrous acid in hydrochloric acid solution at 0-5°0C to form benzene diazonium chloride.

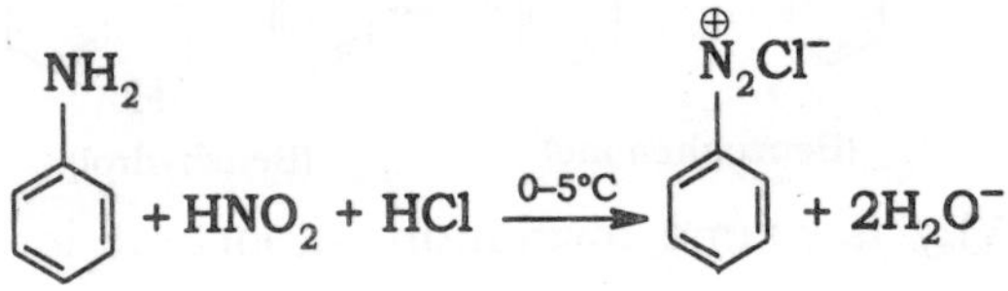

This reaction is called *diazotisation* reaction.

Q.24. Write down the reaction involved in the preparation of sulphanilic acid from aniline.

Ans. Aniline when heated with conc. H_2SO_4 at 180°C forms anilinium hydrogen sulphate, which eliminate a water molecule to form N-phenyl sulphamic acid, which on heating rearranges to sulphanilic acid.

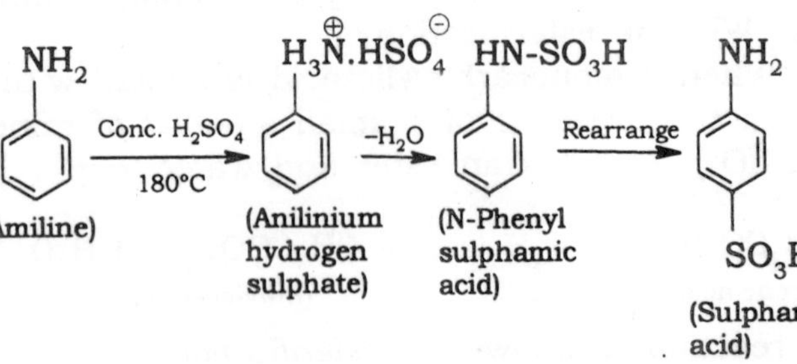

(Amiline) (Anilinium hydrogen sulphate) (N-Phenyl sulphamic acid) (Sulphanilic acid)

Q.25. Explain Beckmann rearrangement.

Ans. When a ketoxime is treated with acidic catalyst such as H_2SO_4, PCl_5, etc. it gets converted into a substituted amide.

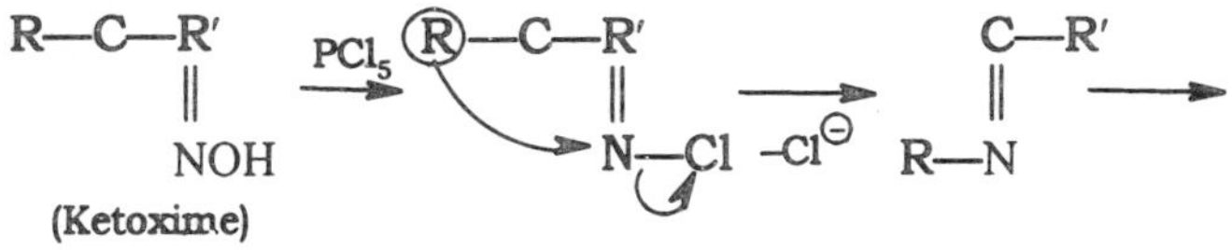

(Ketoxime)

(Where R, R' = Alkyl or anyl group)

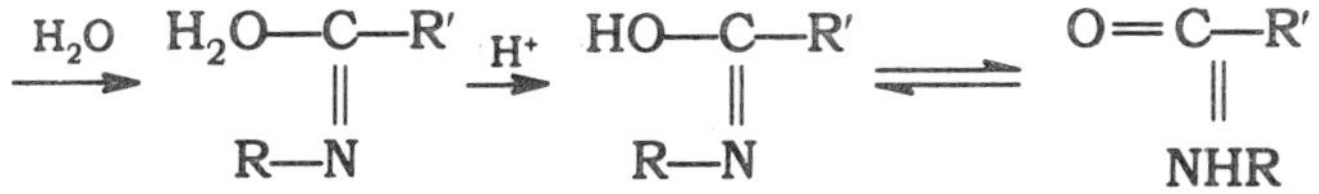

(Amide)

Q.26. Write down the Beckmann rearrangement product of benzophenone oxime in presence of acidic reagents H_2SO_4.

Ans. Beckmann rearrangement product of benzophenone oxime is benzanilide.

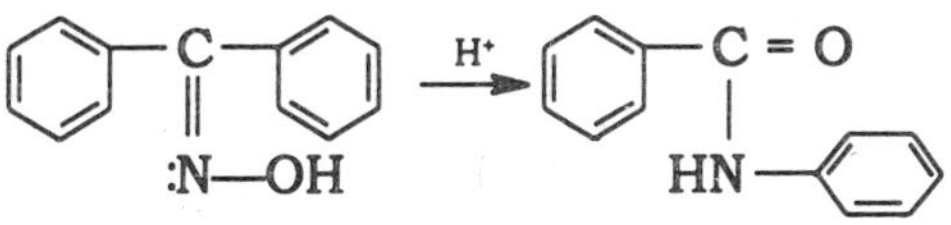

(Benzophenone oxime) (Benzanilide)

Q.27. Explain Fries rearrangement.

Ans. Esters of phenolic compounds on treatment with anhydrous aluminium chloride yields o- and p-hydroxy ketones. This reaction is reffered to as Fries rearrangement, e.g. hydroquinone diacetate on treatment with anhydrous aluminium chloride gives 2, 5 dihydroxy acetophenone.

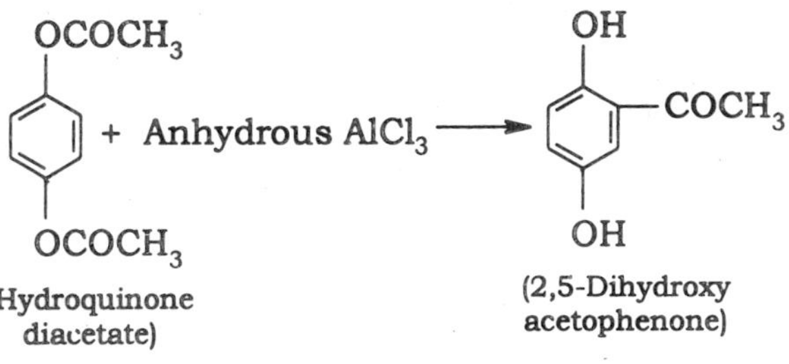

(Hydroquinone diacetate) (2,5-Dihydroxy acetophenone)

Q.28. Bromination of acetanilide gives a mixture of o- and p-bromoacetanilide. How would you obtain only p-product. Why only o- and p-products obtained?

Ans. By crystallization with alcohol. Because o-bromoacetanilide is more soluble in alcohol (ethanol) as compared with p-isomer. —$NHCOCH_3$ is electron donating group and increases the electron density at ortho- and para-positions.

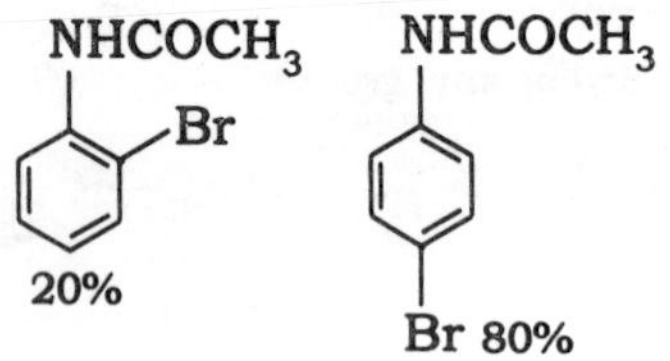

Q.29. What is caffeine?

Ans. Caffeine is a derivative of xanthine. It is 1, 3, 7–trimethylxanthine.

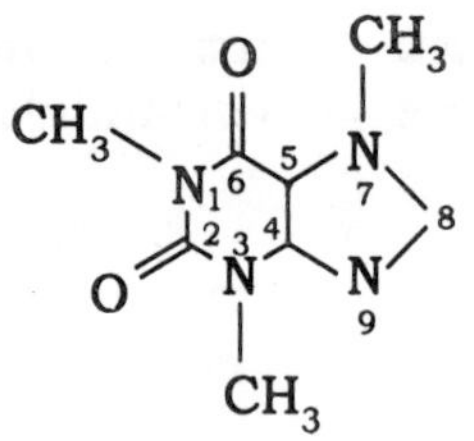

(Caffeine)

Q.30. How would you remove tannins from the aqueous extract of tea leaves?

Ans. Tannins can be removed from the aqueous extract by the addition of a solution of lead acetate. The excess of lead is removed as lead sulphate by the addition of sulphuric acid.

Q.31. Why is activated charcoal added in the process of isolation of caffeine form tea leaves?

Ans. Activated charcoal removes most of the colouring and other extraneous matters.

Q.32. What is casein?

Ans. Casein is a phospho protein composed of at least 15 amino acids. It is principal protein of milk. Cow milk contains about 3% of casein. Pure casein is an amorphous. tasteless, odourless and hygroscopic white solid. It is insoluble in most organic solvent. It is soluble in sodium hydroxide.

Q.33. What is lactose?

Ans. Lactose is a disaccharide sugar soluble in water. It occurs in the milk of all mammals.

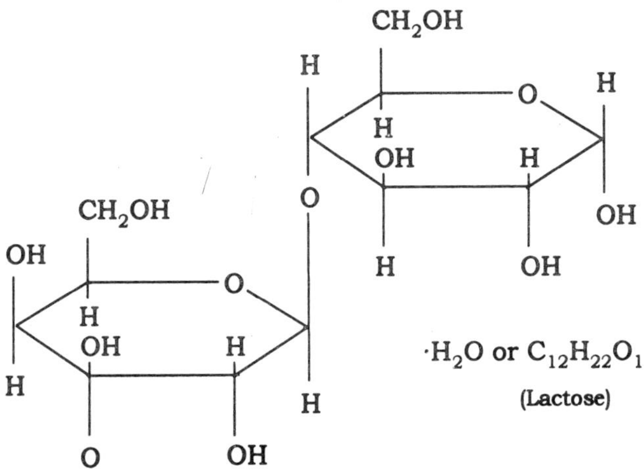

(Lactose)

$\cdot H_2O$ or $C_{12}H_{22}O_{11}\cdot H_2O$

(Lactose)

Reader's Notes

Reader's Notes

Reader's Notes